2/23/11

To Barbara

with best regards,

Phil Coin

# PSYCHIATRY IN INDIANA

## The First 175 Years

Philip M. Coons, M.D., and Elizabeth S. Bowman, M.D.

iUniverse, Inc.
New York   Bloomington

# Psychiatry in Indiana
## The First 175 Years

iUniverse books may be ordered through booksellers or by contacting:

iUniverse
1663 Liberty Drive
Bloomington, IN 47403
www.iuniverse.com
1-800-Authors (1-800-288-4677)

ISBN: 978-1-4502-6072-5 (pbk)
ISBN: 978-1-4502-6074-9 (cloth)
ISBN: 978-1-4502-6073-2 (ebk)

Printed in the United States of America

iUniverse rev. date: 11/16/10

# Dedication

This book is dedicated to the memory of the late William Paul Fisher, M.D., (1929-1998), Professor of Psychiatry at Indiana University School of Medicine. Dr. Fisher nurtured academic excellence, embodied the best of humanity, and instilled in both of us a curiosity about all things psychiatric.

"To study the abnormal is the best way of understanding the normal."

William James

# Contents

## List of Illustrations

# Foreword

I opened the email attachment, clicked the "eco-friendly" setting on the hospital network printer, and picked up the double-sided manuscript on my way out the door from work one day. Having known Drs. Coons and Bowman for nearly twenty-five years, I was confident I would be reading a well-researched, well-documented, thoroughly proofread work, albeit one with the potential for a hint or two of a strong opinion for discerning readers familiar with the authors' professional work and personal beliefs. And indeed, I found it to be just that. I also knew that, as a native of Hendricks County, Indiana, a graduate of the Indiana University School of Medicine and the general psychiatry residency program at the Indiana University Medical Center in Indianapolis, and a former "moonlighter" at Quinco Community Mental Health Center and Bartholomew County Hospital in Columbus and at Central State Hospital in Indianapolis just before it closed, I would find the subject matter of the book to be very interesting, as well as full of nostalgia regarding my Indiana roots.

Yet, I wondered, outside the circle of Indiana psychiatry alums, though not an insignificant number of individuals, who might the readership of this book, be? After reading the manuscript, I am persuaded that this is a book for multiple audiences.

American history buffs will find the links of Indiana state psychiatric hospitals and medical organizations to the role of the federal government, the laws, and the influences of wars, economics, and social and public policy of great interest. Those with a fondness for state and local history will appreciate the descriptions and stories of the old public and private hospitals and how they shaped the identities, cultures, and prosperities of various Hoosier towns and counties. Medical historians with or without a particular interest in psychiatry will see parallels between the coming of age of psychiatry in Indiana and the evolution of general medicine, neurology, neuropsychiatry, pharmacology, and the related fields of medical education, public health, and hospital and medical administration.

Non-physicians in the mental health fields can enjoy this book feeling included and appreciated, for the contributions of many professional disciplines are recounted and honored. Psychologists, chaplains, nurses, social workers, and occupational, physical, and music therapists are but a few of the nonmedical professionals recognized by the authors. Those who labor in health care settings of all kinds, too often unheralded because their vocations are often not counted as professional in nature, can also read this book. The contributions of aides, attendants, kitchen staff, groundskeepers, and other workers to the daily operation of hospitals and care of Indiana's mentally ill are noted throughout the work.

Educators, especially those in special education settings working with individuals with special needs and developmental disabilities, can read this book and be encouraged that public attitudes, laws, policies, and knowledge and multidisciplinary treatment strategies for this population have indeed made progress and advanced over the years. Those with training and interest in the legal profession will enjoy the forensic portions of the book, especially the summaries of landmark cases through the eyes of noted forensic psychiatrist Dr. Philip Coons.

Those of us who attended medical school or trained in psychiatry at the Indiana University Medical Center will be reminded of the landmarks of our professional youth. From the outpatient training clinics in "The Cottages," to the portraits of the grandfathers and grandmothers of Indiana psychiatry hanging in the hallways of Larue Carter Hospital on 10th Street, to the first time one advocated for a patient's best interests before Judge Goodman in the mental health court in Midtown Community Mental Health Center at Wishard Hospital, we are reminded of many key people, places, and experiences in our professional formation.

Most importantly, *Psychiatry in Indiana: The First 175 Years,* reminds us all that individuals and societies are measured not only by how they care for the vulnerable and marginalized in their midst, but how they strive to improve themselves and their treatment of others. Though tragedies and travesties have occurred and must not be forgotten, hopefully the stories of perseverance and improved care for Indiana's psychiatrically ill can encourage and inspire us in our continued efforts in the years to come. Finally, in this book all readers will find the energy and passion for medicine, psychiatry, and excellence in care that Drs. Coons and Bowman have brought not only to Indiana, but to the larger community of students, trainees, colleagues, patients, and their loved ones. Such commitment transcends both time and geographical boundaries.

Mary Lynn Dell, M.D., D.Min.
Associate Professor of Psychiatry, Pediatrics, and Bioethics
Case Western Reserve University School of Medicine, Cleveland, Ohio

# Preface

When we first started writing short articles about the history of psychiatry in Indiana for the *Indiana Psychiatric Society Newsletter,* we never dreamed that one day we would write an entire book on the subject. Yet, history is so interesting and compelling, that we felt that it was a worthwhile task to preserve the history of Indiana psychiatry for future generations.

In *Psychiatry in Indiana: The First 175 Years,* we attempt to cover the era from the time Indiana became a territory in 1800 until about 1975. The senior author (Coons) finished his psychiatry residency in 1975, so that year seemed a logical cutoff point for a number of reasons. First, it's difficult to write about history objectively if one has been a part of it. Second, the rapid gains and numerous changes in psychiatry since 1975 would probably require a second book. A future generation will have to document the story of our era.

This book is primarily about psychiatry and psychiatrists, although to tell an adequate and coherent history of psychiatry in Indiana, we have added considerable information about our professional colleagues, including psychologists, psychiatric social workers, psychiatric nurses, psychiatric attendants, psychiatric researchers, occupational therapists, hospital chaplains, and other physicians and laypersons interested in psychiatry. Psychiatry is a multidisciplinary profession and to ignore these other people would be a disservice to the profession and the field of mental health treatment which we all share.

It was very difficult to decide what to include in this book because of the wealth of material about psychiatry in Indiana. Each chapter in this book could probably have been an entire book. For example, short books or monographs exist for some of Indiana's state hospitals and at least one of state developmental center.

Significant portions of the history of psychiatry in Indiana have been omitted or discussed only briefly. For example, we have chosen to only give examples of community mental health centers and private psychiatric hospitals primarily in central Indiana. We are aware that other midsized cities in Indiana have a rich history of private and community psychiatry, but length considerations prevented us from addressing all of them. In addition we have not written about the history of the treatment of alcohol and drug abuse since substance abuse is not our primary expertise. We have not written about psychiatric self-help groups, such as Alcoholics Anonymous or Recovery, nor have we written about the many wonderful organizations for family members, such as the National Alliance for Mental Illness.

In writing about history, mistakes invariably occur, either because sources contradict one another or we have misunderstood our informants. If we have erred, we deeply regret it and sincerely apologize.

In order to introduce this book to lay readers, our Introduction describes the incredible contributions of psychiatric reformer Dorothea Dix and this is followed in Chapter One by a short history of the diagnosis and treatment of psychiatric illness in the United States. Chapters Two, Three, and Four tell the history of Indiana's public psychiatric hospitals, Chapter Five tells the history of private psychiatric hospitals in central Indiana, and Chapter Six tells the history of Indiana's state developmental centers. Facilities providing psychiatric treatment in correctional settings are discussed in Chapter Seven and Community Mental Health Centers are covered in Chapter Eight. Chapter Nine provides a history of representative psychiatric organizations and Chapter Ten describes the history of the Department of Psychiatry at Indiana University School of Medicine where most Indiana psychiatrists and many other mental health professionals received their training. Child Psychiatry is the focus of Chapter Eleven. Chapters Twelve and Thirteen deal with notable psychiatrists in the Nineteenth and Twentieth Centuries respectively, while Chapter Fourteen deals with notable non-psychiatrists. Chapter Fifteen consists of a potpourri of forensic issues. Chapter Sixteen concludes with an assortment of famous cases culled from books and other media.

# Acknowledgments

There are many individuals and organizations that I [Philip Coons] wish to thank because without their help this book would not have been possible. First and foremost I'd like to thank my wife, Elizabeth Bowman, M.D., who unknowingly started work on this book about twenty-five years ago when she wrote the history of the Indiana Neuro-Psychiatric Association, forerunner of the Indiana Psychiatric Society. Her editorial assistance has been invaluable as has been her forbearance in tolerating my short overnight trips around Indiana to conduct research.

I [Elizabeth Bowman] wish to thank my husband and co-author, Philip Coons, for conducting the background research for this book, for obtaining and cataloguing the photographs therein, and for writing the first draft of most of the chapters. His organizational skills, historical research skills, and perseverance made this book possible.

We wish to thank members of the Indiana Psychiatric Society, who have graciously granted their time for personal interviews about the history of psychiatry in Indiana. Most importantly, we wish to thank the late Drs. Philip Reed and John Greist, Sr., for their interviews with Dr. Bowman in the 1980s about the beginnings of the Indiana Neuro-Psychiatric Association. We are grateful to Drs. Lane Ferree, Sherman Franz, Wesley Kissel, Philip Morton, Alan Schmetzer, Rose Ann Fisher, and Norma French for providing recollections and/or photographs. Last, but not least, we thank Sara Stramel, Executive Director of the Indiana Psychiatric Society, for her assistance.

We appreciate the assistance of Drs. John Nurnberger, Jr., George Parker, and Alan Schmetzer in the Department of Psychiatry at Indiana University School of Medicine. Hugh Hendrie, M.B., Ch.B., former chair of the Department of Psychiatry, and his former administrative assistant, Francine Bray, deserve special mention for preserving the Hugh Hendrie papers in the Archives at Indiana University Purdue University at Indianapolis. Robbie Smith, current administrative assistant to departmental chair Christopher McDougle, M.D., also deserves thanks.

Dwight Schuster, M.D., the Dean of Indiana Psychiatry deserves special thanks for proving us with valuable information about Norways Hospital and the early history of the Psychiatry Department at Methodist Hospital. Joyce Bowman, R.N., who was a nursing student at Norways and then worked at both Richmond State Hospital and Larue Carter Hospital provided much information from a nursing point of view.

Those who consented to individual interviews also deserve special mention because they gave this book a personal side that would otherwise not exist: Vincent Alig, M.D., Joyce Bowman, R.N., Angie Eckstein, M.S.W., Catherine Eversole, M.S.W., the late John Greist, Sr., M.D., Donald Jolly, M.D., Marcia Lurie, O.T.R., Philip Morton, M.D., the late Philip Reed, M.D., Ruth Rogers, M.S.W., Dwight Schuster, M.D., Iver Small, M.D., Joyce Small, M.D., Art Sterne, Ph.D., and Wanda Stoops, M.S.

Individuals on the past and current staff at Indiana's state hospitals and state developmental centers provided an incredible amount of information about the histories of their respective state hospitals. These individuals include Drs. Vincent Alig, Philip Morton, Joyce and Iver Small, Ms Ruth Rogers, and Art Sterne, Ph.D., at Larue Carter Memorial Hospital; Mary Helen Hennessey Nottage and Ann Blank at the Medical History Museum at Central State Hospital; Theresa Arvin and Catherine Eversole at Evansville State Hospital; Shadi Lilly, Brian Newell, and Jacqueline Phillips at Logansport State Hospital; Karen Friedersdorf, Dr. Donna Smith, and Debora Woodfill at Madison State Hospital; Jeff Butler, Donald Graber, M.D., Tara Jamison, and Mary Johnson at Richmond State Hospital; and Angie Eckstein for the Muscatatuck State Developmental Center.

Library archivists including Nancy Eckerman at the Ruth Lilly Medical Library at Indiana University School of Medicine, Brian Moberly at the Indiana University Purdue University Archives in Indianapolis, Ron Grimes at the Jefferson County Historical Society Research Library in Madison, Indiana, and Vicki Casteel and Alan January at the Indiana State Archives were especially helpful as was Judy Smith in the Medical Library at Larue Carter Memorial Hospital.

Rev. Al Galloway was helpful in pointing us towards information about chaplaincy in Indiana's state mental hospitals. The Honorable Judge Evan Goodman, Marion County Courts, provided much needed insight into Indiana's first mental health court.

We wish to thank the staff librarians at the Allen County Public Library in Fort Wayne, Cass County Historical Society in Logansport, Indiana, Evansville Vanderburgh Public Library, Indiana Historical Society, Indiana State Library, Indianapolis Marion County Public Library, Jefferson County Historical Society in Madison, Indiana, Jennings County Public Library in North Vernon, Indiana, Morrison Reeve Library in Richmond, Indiana, New Albany/Floyd Co. Public Library, and the St. Joseph County Public Library.

Finally I [Philip Coons] wish to thank Karen Zack, former Montgomery County, Indiana historian, with whom I share an interest for all things historical. Her mentorship in teaching me how to write about history and make it interesting has been invaluable.

# Introduction

"I come to present the strong claims of suffering humanity. I come to place before the Legislature of Massachusetts the condition of the miserable, the desolate, the outcast. I come as the advocate of helpless, forgotten, insane men and women; of beings sunk to a condition from which the unconcerned world would start with real horror."

Dorothea Dix,
Memorial to the Legislature of Massachusetts,
1843

Prior to the opening of the Indiana Hospital for the Insane in Indianapolis in 1848 the only places where folks with mental illness, feeble-mindedness, and epilepsy were housed, besides being kept at home or in farm buildings, were in county jails and county poor houses. This "poor relief" was part of the criminal justice system until 1936. County jails were usually divided into two sections, one for debtors and one for criminals. The first county poor house was established in 1825 and by 1850 every county had established a poor house. Although the Indiana constitutions of 1816 and 1851 indicated that these facilities were for the aged and infirm, the poor houses, in reality, housed those with mental and developmental disabilities as well as the blind, deaf, and the physically handicapped.[1]

Indiana owes a large debt of gratitude to Dorothea Lynde Dix (1802-1887), American activist for the indigent insane. She was born in Maine and grew up in Massachusetts, but at the age of twelve left her alcoholic and abusive father. A victim of poor health, in her early life she taught in several girls schools and wrote a number of children's stories and books. After spending four years in England, she returned home and over the next decade visited numerous jails, poor houses, and mental institutions all the way from New Hampshire to Louisiana. She published numerous memorials to state legislatures and worked closely with state legislative committees in order to arrange for the construction of state hospitals for the insane. During the Civil War, Ms Dix was appointed superintendent of the Union Army nurses. She made certain that both the Union and Confederate wounded received proper treatment.

In Indiana Ms Dix visited poor houses and jails in many counties. Between August and October of 1847, her findings were published in an eight-part series of articles in the *Indiana State Journal*, a weekly newspaper in Indianapolis.[2]

At the time Ms Dix made her memorial to the Indiana State Legislature in 1848, there existed twenty state hospitals for the insane and several private hospitals in nineteen states. She reported that she had seen nine thousand individuals with insanity, mental deficiency, or epilepsy who were deprived of adequate care and living in jails, poor houses, and private dwellings. She had seen thousands who had been chained up and physically abused. From 1845 until 1847 she traveled the length and breadth of Indiana and found about nine hundred indigent mentally ill. Some were confined in pens without clothing or shelter.

What follows are brief excerpts from her Indiana survey of Indiana jails and poor houses:

> "Marion County Jail at Indianapolis...This jail is very inconvenient and ill planned...It was not in any respect, when I saw it, in order for the reception of prisoners...The Poor-house in Marion County...the whole establishment was clean and carefully managed...The poor were neatly and well clothed."[3]

> "The Jail of Montgomery County, Crawfordsville, is of the worst and most inconvenient construction....I was told that the Grand Jury had more than once, declared this prison a nuisance....The poor house farm of Fountain County...the cabins for the poor, miserable and wholly insufficient for the wants of the inmates...the two insane girls...lodged...on the floor...."[4]

> "Carrol [sic] County Jail...the dungeon on the ground floor, I found dark, dismal and dirty, about fourteen feet square..."[5]

"Allen county jail at Fort Wayne...the prison consists of one dungeon, fourteen feet square, lighted and ventilated by two small windows...I found in it three prisoners, one of whom was insane, and above stairs two others, also insane...the poor-house of Allen...was in a condition very discreditable to the county...There were but three inmates...two old men, and a deaf and dumb boy... who seemed to me partially insane...his passions, quite ungovernable, rendered him a very dangerous inmate."[6]

"The poor in Grant county are sold to the lowest bidder or bidders...There are several insane in the county...but one I saw abroad in a state of excitement coursing up and down through the woods on horseback, shouting, and singing vociferously. I learnt that she had 'not been right for a long while'... Orange County Jail at Paoli, is constructed of timber; it consists of two apartments, not well ventilated, 'may be warmed with charcoal,' a dangerous practice, as it is well known through often fatal results in many places."[7]

"Vanderburgh county poor house and farm...of the five inmates, all were insane or partially so; one was at times furiously excited, so as to render, it was believed, close confinement and chaining necessary."[8]

"Switzerland County Poor-house...in July a blind man and his wife occupied one room, and in this was chained to the floor a furiously excited crazy woman; between who and the other female, said my informant, were 'daily right hard fights' and some who see its shocking exhibition... 'think it excellent fun'..."[9]

Just prior to the Civil War private citizens and volunteer associations were beginning to express dismay over conditions in county homes. In 1844 Indiana opened the Asylum for the Education of the Deaf and Dumb (currently the Indiana School for the Deaf) in Indianapolis. Three years later the Indiana Institute for the Education of the Blind (currently the Indiana School for the Blind) was established in Indianapolis. Shortly thereafter private orphans' homes and county orphanages were established to keep children out of county poor houses.

In 1889 the Indiana State Legislature established the Indiana Board of State Charities to investigate and look after the burgeoning system of public charitable and correctional institutions. Each institution was charged with making an annual report to the state legislature.

# A Brief History of Psychiatry
# in the United States

"It has been remarked, that the maniacs of the male sex in all hospitals, who assist in cutting wood, making fires, and digging in a garden, and the females who are employed in washing, ironing, and scrubbing floors, often recover, while persons, whose rank exempts them from performing such services, languish away their lives within the walls of the hospital."

Benjamin Rush,
*Medical Inquiries and Observations*
*upon the Diseases of the Mind*, 1812

We begin the history of psychiatry in the United States with Benjamin Rush, M.D., (1745-1813), the founder of American psychiatry. Rush was not only a physician but a writer, educator, humanitarian, and signer of the Declaration of Independence. He was the author of the first textbook on psychiatry, *Medical Inquiries and Observations upon the Diseases of the Mind*,[1] first published in 1812. In his book Rush described hypochondriasis, mania, dissociation, and derangements of faith, memory, will, morality, and sexual appetite. Rush's remedies for these various ailments included garlic infusions, blood letting, purging, and the use of bark or opium. Perhaps the most interesting and sometimes appropriate treatments, even by today's standards, are his remedies for an overactive sexual appetite. These included matrimony, avoidance of the opposite sex, avoidance of obscene pictures, temperance with alcohol, cold baths, purges, diets of bread and water, and immersion in business or study.

Another of Rush's accomplishments was a successful campaign to establish a separate ward for mental patients at the Pennsylvania

1

Hospital. Rush was considered a pioneer in occupational therapy because he advocated work for both men and women. He was a pioneer in alcohol addiction treatment and was the first to conceptualize alcoholism as a medical disease rather than a sinful failing. Rush was a prominent educator who trained over three thousand medical students during his lifetime.

Dr. Rush worked at the Pennsylvania Hospital, which opened in Philadelphia in 1751. The hospital's care of the mentally ill in overly crowded psychiatric wards was removed to west Philadelphia in 1841 when the Pennsylvania Hospital for the Insane was opened. The hospital's first superintendent was Thomas Story Kirkbride, M.D., (1809-1883), founder of the American Association of Medical Superintendents of American Institutions for the Insane and also inventor of the Kirkbride Plan of constriction of hospitals for the insane (See Chapter 2). The Pennsylvania Hospital eventually became the Institute of Pennsylvania Hospital. The hospital had some private rooms and the patients not only received medical treatment, but worked outside, participated in recreational activities, attended lectures, and had use of a hospital library.

The Pennsylvania Hospital for the Insane, however, was not the nation's first psychiatric hospital. That honor goes to the Friends Hospital[2] which opened its doors to fifty patients on May 15, 1817. Isaac Bonsall, a successful Pennsylvania farmer, was its first superintendent. The hospital was situated on fifty-eight acres of farmland and the area that wasn't cultivated included a park-like setting with shaded walks, ponds, and forest paths. This hospital, operated by the Quakers, was a haven for the insane. In order to maximize light and fresh air, rooms were placed on only one side of a corridor. Males were quartered on one end of the hospital and women on the other. The more violent patients were housed on the second floor and there were special rooms on the fourth floor for "noisy" patients. Patients were helped to recover from their illnesses by working on the hospital grounds and farm. They were treated humanely and were part of a family, which included the superintendent and his family, physicians, a matron, a nurse, and attendants. The symptoms of mental illness requiring treatment were like those encountered at the Indiana Hospital for the Insane (See Chapter 2), including melancholy, abusive behavior, filthiness, negativism, agitation, depression, suicidal behavior, self-mutilation, anxiety, suspicion, insomnia, excitement, anorexia, alcohol and drug addiction, and "obliterated ideas."

Early insane asylums in the United States and elsewhere operated under the principles of "moral treatment" or "traitement moral" as coined by Philippe Pinel (1745-1826), the famous French physician who unchained patients at the hospital Bicêtre in Paris, France. The moral approach involved treating patients humanely, without restraint, with close patient-staff interaction, and involving them in various therapeutic activities.

The first association of physicians treating mental disorders was called the American Association of Medical Superintendents of American Institutions for the Insane. This group of thirteen superintendents of American insane asylums first met in Philadelphia in October 1844. It was the first medical specialty group in the United States and it collected statistical data about mental illness and furthered the treatment of the insane. It 1892 this association's name was changed to the American Medico-Psychological Association to allow assistant physicians working in state insane asylums to become members. Finally in 1921 the group's name was changed to its present form, the American Psychiatric Association.

The classification of psychiatric illnesses has a long history. Hippocrates, the famous Greek physician who lived during the fourth century BCE, and his followers were the first to classify physical and mental illnesses. Hippocrates thought that illnesses were due to an imbalance in blood, yellow bile, black bile, and phlegm. The words mania, melancholia, paranoia, and phobia actually stem from the Greek. For example, Hippocrates thought that melancholia was caused by an excess of black bile. English physician, Thomas Sydenham (1624-1689), developed the concept of a syndrome, or a collection of symptoms which made an illness. During the eighteenth century the classification of physical and mental diseases, developed from the idea of biological taxonomy, developed by Carl Linneaus (1707-1778). The taxonomy approach was abandoned in the nineteenth century in favor anatomical and clinically descriptive approaches. It wasn't until the late nineteenth century that German psychiatrist Emil Kraepelin (1856-1926), divided the psychoses into manic depression and dementia praecox, which was later to become known as schizophrenia, a term coined by Swiss psychiatrist Eugen Bleuler (1857-1939). It was left up to Sigmund Freud (1856-1939) to describe the various neuroses. Finally, the mid-twentieth century saw the publication of the first *Diagnostic and Statistical Manual of Mental Disorders* by the American Psychiatric Association in 1952.[3]

Isaac Ray (1807-1881), American psychiatrist and founding member of the American Association of Medical Superintendents of American Institutions for the Insane, is credited with originating American forensic psychiatry. In 1838 he published *"A Treatise on the Medical Jurisprudence of Insanity,"*[4] an authoritative text for many years. This text was used extensively by defense attorney, Sir Alexander Cockburn, in his defense of Daniel M'Naghten at his 1843 trial for the murder of Edward Drummond, the private secretary of England's Prime Minister, Robert Peel. Out of this trial grew the M'Naghten Rule, whereby an accused is judged not guilty by reason of insanity.

In addition to the development of moral treatment of the nineteenth century, a number of other psychiatric treatments evolved during the first half of the twentieth century. Various types of the "water cure" have been with us since antiquity, but hydrotherapy as a psychiatric treatment was a late nineteenth and early twentieth century phenomenon. Emil Kraepelin first wrote about the benefits of long baths for dementia patients in 1891. By the mid 1930s all state psychiatric hospitals had hydrotherapy units. A typical hydrotherapy unit consisted of a room filled with special bath tubs. The patient's body was submersed in a tub of warm water and a canvas sheet with a hole for the patient's head and neck was stretched over the tub. The warm water was continuously flowing and was set at a temperature, usually between ninety five and one hundred degrees Fahrenheit, ordered by the physician. This form of hydrotherapy was supposed to exert a calming effect on the agitated patient. A similar form of therapy was called a hot or cold wet sheet pack or wrap. In this form of therapy the patient was wrapped in a sheet which ranged in temperature from forty to one hundred degrees Fahrenheit. Generally agitated patients were wrapped in cold sheets. Sheets were cooled by either placing them in a tub of ice water or placing them in a freezer.[5-7]

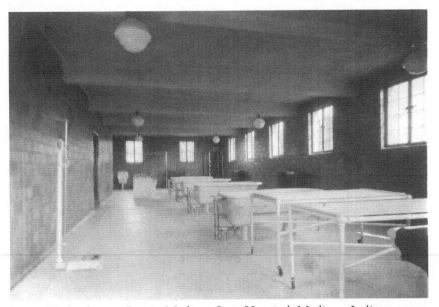

Hydrotherapy Room, Madison State Hospital, Madison, Indiana

In 1917 Julius von Wagner-Jauregg, M.D., (1857-1940), an Austrian physician, discovered the "fever cure" for tertiary neurosyphilis, a frequent cause of mental illness until penicillin was discovered. In this form of therapy the patient was infected with malaria. The infection caused recurrent fevers, which in turn resulted in a dramatic improvement in patients with neurosyphilis. This form of treatment was eventually adapted for use at Central State Hospital in Indiana. In 1927 Wagner-Jauregg became the first psychiatrist to ever win the Nobel Prize.

Another Austrian psychiatrist Manifred Sakel, M.D., (1900-1957), invented insulin coma therapy in 1927. In this form of therapy, a coma from low blood sugar was induced through the injection of insulin. Such treatments sometimes brought about dramatic improvements in schizophrenic patients. This treatment was dangerous, however, and was abandoned with the introduction of Thorazine, the first antipsychotic medication. Insulin coma therapy was used extensively in Indiana mental institutions.

Hungarian neuropsychiatrist Ladislas Meduna, M.D., (1896-1964), invented Metrazol shock therapy in 1934. In this form of therapy pentylenetetrazol was injected to induce seizures. This form of therapy produced dramatic improvements in schizophrenic patients who were in a catatonic state, an extreme form of motor rigidity which the patient may hold a posture without moving for hours or days. This form of therapy was also used in many psychiatric hospitals in Indiana.

In 1938, electroconvulsive therapy was invented by Ugo Cerletti, M.D., (1877-1963) and Lucio Bini, M.D., (1908-1964), both Italian psychiatrists. In this type of treatment an electric current is applied to the head in order to induce an electrical seizure. Electroconvulsive therapy was used initially in schizophrenia and later in those with either depression or mania. Although it has largely been abandoned in the treatment of schizophrenia in favor of medication, it still has a major role in treating severe depression or mania which has not responded to medication and psychotherapy.

Egas Moniz, M.D., (1874-1955), a Portuguese neurologist, was the developer of cerebral leucotomy or lobotomy, an early form of psychosurgery, in which the connections of the prefrontal cortex are separated from the frontal lobe of the brain. In the mid-1930s Moniz and neurosurgeon, Pedro Lima, M.D., perfected their technique. It had been known for many years that disease of the prefrontal areas of the brain resulted in a calm, sometimes apathetic state. In their initial study of twenty-two patients, composed mostly of schizophrenics and depressed patients, Moniz and Lima noted that two thirds of patients who underwent lobotomy were either greatly or moderately improved in their anxiety and agitation. Walter Freeman, M.D., (1895-1972), an American neurologist, became fascinated with Moniz's work, and together with James Watts, M.D., (1904-1994), an American neurosurgeon, brought this surgical technique to the United States. Dr. Freeman, however, became dissatisfied with the laborious neurosurgical technique and developed the trans-orbital lobotomy whereby an ice pick-like devise was driven by means of a mallet over the eyeball and through the upper part of the eye socket. This instrument was then swept side to side in order to sever the prefrontal fibers from the rest of the frontal lobe. Dr. Watts was aghast when he discovered Freeman performing this procedure in their office and their partnership abruptly ended. Freeman went on, however, to demonstrate this procedure in mental hospitals across the United States. By 1951 nearly nineteen thousand patients had been lobotomized in the United States. Perhaps the most famous patient to undergo a trans-orbital lobotomy was Rosemary Kennedy, sister to President John F. Kennedy.[8] Lobotomies were performed at two state mental hospitals in Indiana, Logansport State Hospital and Evansville State Hospital.

In 1938 Donnadieu first reported atropine coma therapy. Atropine coma therapy was used for treating agitation experienced during psychoses.

This form of treatment consisted of the induction of a prolonged four to ten-hour coma by the intramuscular injection, intravenous injection, or even intra-carotid injection of massive doses (150-200 mg) of atropine. Although sedatives were given before such treatments, this type of treatment never became wildly popular with patients because of the disorientation, delirium, hallucinations, rapid heart rate, and nausea and vomiting caused by the atropine. These treatments were labor intensive because of the extensive pretreatment medical workups and extensive medical monitoring required during the duration of the coma. The usual course of treatment consisted of five to twenty-five treatments given two to six times a week. By 1958 Forrer and Miller reported that they were able to terminate the atropine coma with physostigmine. Side effects of atropine coma therapy included urinary retention and hyperthermia. Mortality ranged from none in one large series of three thousand patients to one in four hundred patients. Atropine coma therapy never gained wide acceptance in the United States and was mostly used in a few state hospitals from about 1950 through about 1970.[9, 10] Evansville State Hospital used atropine coma therapy.

These crude somatic treatments came to an abrupt end, however, when Thorazine was brought to the United States in the mid-1950s. Thorazine, or chlorpromazine hydrochloride, was first synthesized in France in 1950 and the first published clinical trial was performed in Paris in 1952 by Drs. Jean Delay and Pierre Deniker, both French psychiatrists. Chlorpromazine was first marked in Europe as Largactil. It and other similar antipsychotic medications revolutionized the treatment of schizophrenia and enabled many long-term patients with schizophrenia to be released from state psychiatric hospitals.

In 1948 John Cade, M.D., (1912-1980), an Australian psychiatrist, discovered that lithium carbonate an oxidized salt of the metal lithium, stabilized the mood of those suffering from manic depression, now known as bipolar disorder. Mogens Shou, M.D., (1918-2005), a Danish psychiatrist replicated Cade's results in a double-blind study published in 1954. By the mid-1960s lithium carbonate was in wide use in the United States. It was the first pharmacologic agent to effectively treat both the mania and depression of bipolar disorder. A research group at Larue Carter Memorial Hospital was involved in the early testing of lithium carbonate in the United States.

While the early somatic treatments developed in the late nineteenth and early twentieth centuries in the United States and Europe, a revolution in thinking about the psyche was brewing in Austria, Germany, and Great Britain. Sigmund Freud, M.D., (1856-1939), an Austrian neurologist, was a leading proponent of talk therapy. Through his theories about the unconscious, defense mechanisms, psychosexual development, the structure of the psyche, and his therapeutic concepts including free association and transference, Freud founded the psychoanalytic school of psychiatry. In September 1909 Freud came to the United States and lectured at Clark University in Worcester, Massachusetts. Freud's youngest child, Anna Freud (1895-1982), along with Austrian-born British psychoanalyst Melanie Klein (1882-1969), were cofounders of psychoanalytic child psychiatry. The accomplishments of these pioneers and their followers form the basis for most of our modern ideas about adult and child psychotherapy. Psychoanalytic training centers were established in the United States, initially mostly on the East Coast. Two such centers, in Chicago and Cincinnati, lay just outside Indiana's borders. Indiana narrowly missed out on having a psychoanalytic treatment center when Herbert Gaskill, M.D., chairman of the Indiana University School of Medicine Department of Psychiatry, left Indianapolis and moved to Denver Colorado where he established the Colorado Psychoanalytic Institute.

Lightner Witmer, Ph.D., (1867-1956) was the founder of the first outpatient psychological clinic at the University of Pennsylvania in 1896. He is regarded as the founder of clinical psychology and he, along with Stanley Hall, Ph.D., (1844-1924), founded the American Psychological Association in 1892. The founding of child guidance clinics in the United States was not far behind. The first was opened in Chicago in 1909 just ten years after the first juvenile court opened there in 1899. The first training program in child psychiatry began at the Illinois Juvenile Psychopathic Institute in Chicago in 1917.[11] The establishment of child guidance clinics in Indiana is discussed in Chapter 11.

Further history about the Indiana insane asylums can be found in Chapters 2, 3, and 4 and the history of community mental health centers can be found in Chapter 8. For an in-depth, but somewhat cynical, study of two early nineteenth-century psychiatric hospitals in New York see Ellen Dwyer's, *Homes for the mad: Life inside two nineteenth-century asylums.*[12]

CHAPTER 2

# Public Psychiatric Institutions

"Be it enacted by the General Assembly of the State of
Indiana, that John Evans, Livingston Dunlap, and James
Blake, be, and they are hereby appointed a board of
commissioners to select and purchase such a tract of land,
not exceeding two hundred acres in quantity, as may be
most suitable, in regard to health and convenience, for the
location of a State lunatic asylum."

*General Laws of the State of Indiana passed at the twenty-*
*ninth session of the General Assembly begun on the first*
*Monday in December 1944.* Indianapolis, Indiana: J.P.
Chapman, 1845.

### Historical Overview

In the next three chapters are descriptions of Indiana's adult public
psychiatric institutions including Central State Hospital (now closed),
Evansville State Hospital, Larue Carter Memorial Hospital, Logansport
State Hospital, Madison State Hospital, and Richmond State Hospital.

The history of Indiana's state psychiatric facilities illustrates national
trends in mental health care observed across the United States. The
enrollment in Indiana's psychiatric institutions declined dramatically
during the twentieth century due to the introduction of antipsychotic
medication and the move towards community care. For example, in the
1939-40 fiscal year the average daily census at the five state hospitals,
excluding Carter Hospital, which had not been built yet, was 8,323
patients.[1] During the 2007-08 fiscal year the average daily population
for five state hospitals, excluding Central State Hospital, which had been
closed, was 1,100 patients.[2]

Over the years Indiana's state mental hospitals have received much criticism, some well-deserved and some not. As pointed out under the section on Central State Hospital, criticism often ran in cycles; a period of legislative neglect was usually followed by a period of legislative concern where more monies were made available to operate the state hospitals.

One such period of neglect occurred during the years preceding and during World War II when most psychiatric physicians were away serving in the military and most of our national effort and money was dedicated towards providing for our men and women in uniform. In the years immediately following World War II there was a nationwide outcry against the "Bedlams" that we had created through neglect. *Life Magazine* ran an investigative article in 1946 which exposed our nation's disgrace.[3] In 1946 the total population of the one hundred eighty state mental institutions stood at four hundred thousand. Patient abuse was said to be rampant. Diets were poor. Restraints were overused. The institutions were woefully understaffed with underpaid personnel. There was overcrowding. Not all physicians were competent. In Ohio patients were being treated for $1.20 a day in their state psychiatric institutions. Amazingly much of this institutional neglect came to light through the efforts and surveys of conscientious objectors who had worked as attendants in state hospitals during World War II.

Five years after the first *Life Magazine* article, its author, Albert Maisel, wrote a follow-up piece.[4] What Maisel found was quite different. The aroused public indignation had brought real reform. Legislators appropriated more money making it easier to hire the cadre of doctors, nurses, and attendants that staffed the large state hospitals. Monetary appropriations and state hospital staff nationwide had increased by one hundred percent. The number of physicians grew by nineteen percent and graduate nurses by thirty-five percent. State hospital social workers and occupational therapists had doubled in numbers and psychologists had tripled.

One success story mentioned by Maisel was Logansport State Hospital, which had hired John A. Larson, M.D., as its new superintendent. Physician staff increased from three to ten and graduate nurses from six to sixteen. Student nurses were brought in to help. An eight-hour work day was instituted for attendants and attendants were provided training courses. The attendant staff increased from 178 to 252. Volunteers were recruited. Restraints were abolished except for the immediate post-operative period. These efforts resulted in the discharge and admission rates nearly doubling.

## Hospital Construction

Early nineteenth century public insane asylum construction in the United States followed two architectural plans for large state psychiatric institutions, the "Kirkbride Plan" and the "Cottage Plan." Indiana was part of this trend.

The Women's Building at Central State Hospital was constructed according to the Kirkbride Plan. This plan was developed by Thomas Story Kirkbride (1809-1883), a Philadelphia psychiatrist and one of the founders of the Association of Medical Superintendents of American Institutions for the Insane, forerunner of the American Psychiatric Association. Kirkbride wrote an influential book in which he espoused an architectural style for hospitals for the insane.[1] At Central State Hospital the Kirkbride Plan of the Women's Building provided for the construction of a very large, three to five story, Victorian-style hospital building in which the administration section was front and center and the numerous patient wards were staggered out and behind. This design made for well-lit and well-ventilated hospital wards. The square footage of the Women's Building totaled 337,234.

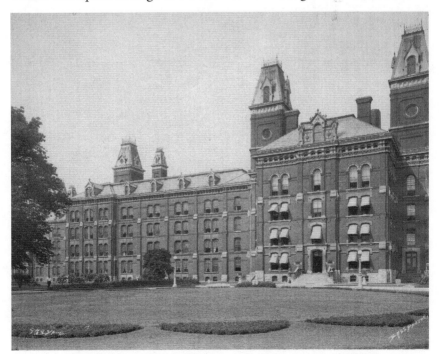

Women's Building, Central State Hospital, Indianapolis,
Indiana, photo courtesy of Indiana Historical Society

Both Madison State Hospital and Logansport State Hospital were built according to the Cottage Plan. This concept of construction was a radical departure from the massive buildings built according to the nineteenth century Kirkbride Plan. The Cottage Plan involved the construction of a number of smaller buildings, which housed patients and which were grouped around a central administration/services building. Each cottage held between twenty-five to seventy-five patients. One advantage of this type of arrangement of hospital buildings was in fire prevention or control. If one cottage burned it was better than having an entire hospital go up in flames as happened at Evansville State Hospital in 1943.

## Central State Hospital

In 1827 the Indiana State Legislature set aside "square 22," a small parcel of land for the use as a "lunatic asylum" in Indianapolis. Although a hospital was not built here, a log cabin on that site was used as a "crazy house."[1] In 1841, believing that "the state should take care of the mute, the blind, and the insane," a small society was formed in Attica, Indiana.[2] Its members consisted of John Evans, M.D., Isaac Fisher, M.D., Edward Hannigan, and Caleb Jones, M.D. In 1845 Dorothea Dix visited the Indiana General Assembly and motivated them to create the first state hospital in Indiana. The General Assembly passed an act which provided for the purchase of land for a "state lunatic asylum." John Evans, M.D., already a fierce advocate for the mentally ill, recommended that the one hundred sixty acre Bolton farm on the west side of Indianapolis be utilized as the hospital's site. This land was bought at a cost of about fifty-three dollars an acre.[3]

Central State Hospital first opened as the Indiana Hospital for the Insane in Indianapolis on November 21, 1848. On that day the first eight patients were admitted. Dr. R.J. Patterson was the hospital's first superintendent. In its first eleven years of existence Central State Hospital admitted about 1,750 patients. Their occupations were diverse, ranging from physicians to blacksmiths to milliners. The probable causes of insanity listed in the annual report of 1859 include such diverse causes as religious excitement, disappointment in love, spiritual rappings, masturbation, suppression of menses, jealousy, dissipation, dyspepsia, fright, excessive lactation, excessive use of quinine, Mexican War excitement, husbands in California, know-nothingism, mesmerism, reading vile books, political excitement, dissipation, avarice, adultery, and gormandizing, as well as the usual physical causes such as epilepsy, drug and alcohol use, and head injury.[4-5]

The hospital's annual report of 1851 indicated that there were thirteen male and one female masturbators in the hospital. These individuals were seen as shy, nervous, unhappy, remorseful but unable to control their habit, and religiously anxious. Treatment of masturbation consisted of the use of mechanical restraints and aphrodisiacs including conium, camphor, and belladonna. Blisters and cold baths were also prescribed.[2]

Over the years the structures at Central State Hospital changed dramatically. "Old Main," the men's department building was constructed in the late 1840s and was razed in 1941. The most famous building was the Women's Building which was constructed between 1875 and 1878. It had seven large steeples and the hospital became affectionately known to the local populace as "Seven Steeples."[6] By 1964 this building had seriously deteriorated according to then superintendent Clifford L. Williams. Patient rooms had no lights. One bathtub and three toilets served each of the building's twenty-four wards which contained thirty-eight to fifty-five patients each.[7] A new Bahr Treatment Center served as an intensive treatment unit for entering patients.

The hospital became a city to itself. By 1904 it had its own waterworks, power plant, police force, fire department, carpenter shop, cold storage plant, amusement hall, and greenhouse, which raised many plants and shrubs which beautified the grounds.[8] Other structures included an administration building, Men's Building, Women's Building, hospital with operating rooms, bakery, storage buildings, laundry, kitchens, and pathology building.

The Pathology Building has been turned into a medical museum. In its restored condition, it appears much as it did when it was constructed in 1895. Its centerpiece is its lecture hall which is illuminated by skylights. Rows of cane-bottomed chairs rise in a semicircular fashion to fill its two-story extent. Portraits of famous physicians line its walls. Charles Bonsett, M.D, an Indiana University School of Medicine neurologist, was responsible for saving this architectural wonder and turning it into a museum. Until 1956 Indiana University School of Medicine used the building to teach medical students psychiatry. Other rooms in the building contain a funeral parlor, morgue, autopsy room, library, clinical laboratories, photography studio, and physician's offices. The laboratories, which look much as they did in the early 1900s, continued to be operative until the 1960s. The library contains numerous rare medical textbooks.

Still surviving are patient autopsy records, tissue slides, and pathological specimens, mostly brains.[9, 10]

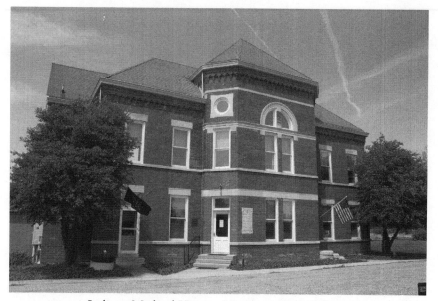

Indiana Medical History Museum, Central State
Hospital, Indianapolis, Indiana

In 1883 William Fletcher, M.D., was made hospital superintendent. In his four years as superintendent he made numerous changes at the hospital including reducing the hospital's medicinal use of whiskey from three gallons to one pint a day, supplying beer to increase appetite in some patients, stopping the secret burial of patients who died while hospitalized, abolishment of the use of restraints, the hiring of the first female physician Sarah Stockton, M.D., instituting a school system, and providing dental care. George Edenharter, M.D., became superintendent in 1893 and continued in this position until his death in 1923. Max Bahr, M.D., followed as superintendent from 1923 until he retired in 1952. During Dr. Bahr's tenure, the malarial treatment of general paresis was pioneered in Indiana and rheumatic brain disease was thought to be a factor in the causation of schizophrenia. See Chapters 12 and 13 for more on the lives of these notable psychiatrists.

One of Dr. Bahr's many accomplishments as superintendent of Central State Hospital was the institution of recreational and occupational therapy. It was thought that the wandering attention of the insane could be trained to concentrate on the many occupational and recreational tasks so as to crowd out of the mind the patient's hallucinatory and delusional thoughts and perceptions. Rug weaving, sewing, basket making, woodworking, and printing were popular occupational therapies and motion pictures, checkers, pool, basketball, croquet, and tennis were favored recreations. These therapies were specifically tailored to meets the needs of patients who had manic depressive psychosis, schizophrenia, paranoia, and general paresis.[11]

Central State Hospital as a large nineteenth century complex which housed several thousand patients at one time has not been immune to criticism. In fact, as one of Indiana's largest psychiatric institutions in the capital city of Indianapolis, it was at the center of controversy in nearly every decade for nearly a century and a half. In a very interesting study, Hugh Hendrie, M.B., Ch.B., former chair of the Department of Psychiatry at Indiana University School of Medicine, and his research assistant Michele Rudnick, did a newspaper search of Indianapolis newspapers from 1900 through 1975. Their paper reports the results of a very complete search of newspapers from 1940 onward. They found that about every five to eight years there was a flurry of newspaper articles that were highly critical of conditions at Central State Hospital. These articles generally continued over two or three years and were followed by a quiescent period of several years, during which many of the articles were benign and or complimentary towards the conditions at Central. Over time the abuse cited included unclean rooms, physical and verbal abuse of patients, patient suicides, inadequate nursing staff, too few psychiatrists, beatings, poor administration, patients dying in accidents, rapes, infestation of rats, and patients lying naked amongst their excrement.[12]

Quoting Alexander Johnson who wrote *Adventures in Social Welfare* in 1923, Hazelrigg writes that conditions were so bad at Central State Hospital in 1888 that Benjamin Harrison, the Republican candidate for president, won the presidency in a very tight presidential race with Grover Cleveland, the Democratic candidate. A corruption investigation in 1877 had uncovered fraud, conspiracies, and abuse of patients at Central State Hospital. This scandal resulted in the creation of the Indiana State Board of Charities to oversee the operation of mental hospitals in Indiana. It also caused the replacement of William Fletcher, M.D., who had instituted many reforms in the previous few years as hospital superintendent.

Having watched from the sidelines the various scandals which have plagued Central State over the years, it is our opinion that the fault for the sometimes deplorable conditions which infest the various state hospitals from time to time really lies with the Indiana State Legislature. It appears that scandals about deplorable conditions goad the legislature into appropriating enough money to better conditions for a time. During the subsequent period of relative calm, less money is appropriated for adequate care. Then the cycle repeats itself. This cycle appears independent of which political party is in power. These ideas are in agreement with Ellen Dwyer who argues that Indiana's fiscal conservatism has undercut the humanitarian goals of state hospitalization for the mentally ill by forcing state hospitals to participate in overcrowding.[13]

Central State Hospital was closed by then Governor Evan Bayh in 1994. Its closure was brought about by media criticism of a series of deaths at Central, fiscal conservatism, and misguided beliefs about the superiority of community care. The controversies about Central State did not immediately end with its closing. Many patients and their families were unhappy about having to go elsewhere for treatment. In a follow-up study of patients who left Central State during its closure, only forty-six percent ended up at home, group homes, or semi-independent living situations. Forty-one percent went to other hospitals or state operated facilities, two percent went to correctional facilities, eight percent went to nursing homes, and about five percent died.[14]

One of the more interesting studies about patients hospitalized at Central State there was published in 1997. Eric T. Dean, Jr., an Indiana attorney, with a Ph.D. in history, published his study, *"Shook Over Hell,"* about PTSD and the Civil War veterans hospitalized at Central State Hospital.[15] Dr. Dean studied pension records and the psychiatric records of 291 Civil War veterans who were hospitalized at the Indiana Hospital of the Insane. His documentation of symptoms of post traumatic stress disorder in Civil War veterans was a milestone in the study of post traumatic stress disorder.

As in many state hospitals patients who died at Central State Hospital, and whose families could not afford burial, were buried on the hospital grounds. The original cemetery at Central was in the northwest section of the hospital grounds near the intersection of Tibbs Avenue and Vermont Street. No markers exist here at this time. A later cemetery, begun in 1905, containing sections two, three, and four, is on the west side of Tibbs Avenue just south of the Mount Jackson Cemetery near the intersection with Washington Street. Records of patient burials are maintained at the Indiana Medical History Museum and the Indiana State Archives.[16]

When Central State Hospital closed in 1994 the remaining staff merged with the staff at Carter Hospital. This resulted in the layoffs of a significant number of Carter staff due to the seniority of Central State employees. At present the only remaining active functions on the Central State Hospital grounds are the Indiana Museum of Medical History, Max Bahr Municipal Park, Indianapolis Fire Department No. 18, and the Indianapolis Metropolitan Police Department's Mounted Patrol stables.

The superintendents of Central State Hospital from 1847 to 1974 include:

| | |
|---|---|
| John Evans, M.D. | 1847 |
| Richard J. Patterson, M.D. | 1848-1853 |
| James S. Athon, M.D. | 1853-1861 |
| James H. Woodburn, M.D. | 1861-1865 |
| Wilson Lockhart, M.D. | 1865-1869 |
| Orpheus Everts, M.D. | 1869-1879 |
| Joseph G. Rogers, M.D. | 1879-1883 |
| William B. Fletcher, M.D. | 1883-1887 |
| Thomas S. Galbraith, M.D. | 1887-1889 |
| Charles E. Wright, M.D. | 1889-1893 |
| George F. Edenharter, M.D. | 1893-1923 |
| Max A. Bahr, M.D. | 1923-1952 |
| Clifford L. Williams, M.D. | 1952-1966 |
| John U. Keating, M.D. | 1966-1974 |

## CHAPTER 3

# Indiana's Public Psychiatric Hospitals Built in the Late Nineteenth Century

"Evansville, Ind., October 24, 1890

Dear Sir – I hereby notify you that this hospital will be opened for patents on the 30th of this month...At the present time I will take two patients from your county – one man and one woman...At present I will take no epileptics...Select from the poor house the patients which you think need care in this institution...Do not send the sick, infirm, bed-ridden or paralytic. It is the unmanageable class that we wish to take first...I would ask you to have the country physician in charge of the poor house to make out a descriptive list of all insane inmates of the poor house and jail...

Very truly yours,
A.J. Thomas
Medical Superintendent"
The insane asylum. To be opened for patients on Thursday next.

*Evansville Journal*, October 26, 1890

## Logansport State Hospital

The Northern Indiana Hospital for the Insane, Indiana's second state mental hospital opened on July 1, 1888. The hospital was nicknamed Longcliff because it was built on a bluff overlooking the Wabash River. The "cliff" is actually a rock outcropping about fifteen feet high. The hospital was built in Logansport, Indiana using the cottage plan on 281 acres of farmland. One hundred sixty acres were purchased from the Andrew Shanklin family and the other 121 acres were donated by the citizens of Cass County. Initial construction provided for an administration building flanked by a number of smaller cottages.

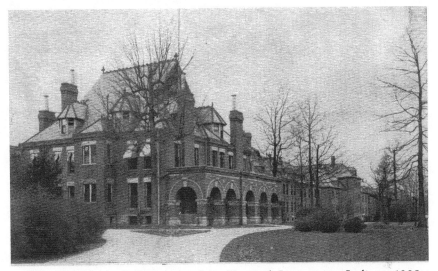

Admission Building, Logansport State Hospital, Logansport, Indiana, 1908

In back of these buildings were a boiler house, pump house, and laundry. Men and women patients were separated into two housing divisions. Additions to the hospital included an auditorium in 1893, a central dining hall in 1896, and additional patient buildings in 1900, by which time the patient population was 731. A pathology building containing a laboratory, morgue, pharmacy and dental office was completed in 1911. In 1930 a separate hydrotherapy department was established. By 1938 the patient population had grown to sixteen hundred. During the 1930s additional buildings were built by the Works Progress Administration to house patients since overcrowding had become such a problem that a "tent camp" had been established for male patients. In 1940 the Men's and Women's Ward Buildings were opened as was the personnel building intended to house employees. Finally in 1940, a nursing department was established, and, due to new treatment practices, time in restraints decreased from 43,512 hours in October 1939 to 5,135 hours in April 1940. By the end of 1940 bed capacity was 2,383 making Logansport State Hospital the largest mental hospital in Indiana. In 1952 an electroencephalographic laboratory was opened and in 1954 the rehabilitation of alcoholic patients began.[1-5]

Salaries were low at the turn of the century. Attendants worked twelve-hour shifts, seven days a week and were paid $30 a month. In 1905 the attendants submitted a petition to have one day off a month and this request was granted. During World War I there was a nearly two hundred percent turnover in staff due to low wages. By the late 1920s the salary of a male attendant was forty dollars a month and female attendants were paid thirty-five dollars a month. By this time attendants had about three days off each month. There was an acute shortage of employees during World War II. By 1945 the shortage was so acute that two to seven wards were without attendants and patients were put in charge of some wards. With the hiring of John Larson, M.D., as superintendent, the hospital began a dramatic turnaround. He established the first art therapy, music therapy, and psychology departments as well as the first psychiatric nursing program in Indiana. He hired the first state hospital chaplain and set up a fire department. By 1956 a forty-hour work week had been established for attendants with a starting monthly salary of $205.[6-8]

The social service department was established in 1941 with Lucy Washbon as the first social worker. In 1949 superintendent John Larson, M.D. expanded the social service program with the help of social service director Murial Youger.[9] The music therapy department was established in 1951 under the direction of Pat Otto.[10]

In addition to staff shortages, several other crises have plagued Logansport State Hospital through the years. On April 19, 1899 a male patient developed smallpox. Superintendent Joseph Rogers, M.D., acted quickly to establish an isolation hospital in two large tents one mile removed from the hospital. The tent was staffed with two volunteers and contained everything necessary for that patient's care including bedding, cook stoves, cooking utensils, lanterns, and medical equipment. The sick male patient had been vaccinated and his illness was mild. A possible epidemic was thus averted through quick action.[11] During a drought in the summer of 1888, water had to be obtained from two springs under the cliff and brought up the hill by a procession of patients and attendants. Over the next several years a number of wells were dug to alleviate the water shortage. It wasn't until 1951 that a modern water works was completed.[12] In July of 1936 Indiana was beset with a terrible heat wave. Between July 4 and July 27 there were fourteen days with temperatures over one hundred degrees Fahrenheit with a range from one hundred to one hundred and eleven degrees Fahrenheit.[13] This merciless heat wave was blamed for the deaths of at least nine patients at the hospital with another six within Cass County.[14] A number of fires have occurred over the years at the hospital including a series of ward fires started by hospital employee Maude Ott in 1944 (See Chapter 16).[15]

Like many late nineteenth century state psychiatric hospitals, Logansport State Hospital was built to be a self-sufficient facility. Its farm raised dairy cattle, pigs, chicken, turkeys, rabbits, ducks, and numerous fruits and vegetables. During one year in the 1940s the hospital produced 178,000 tomato plants and 272,960 cabbage plants. At one time the hospital even had a cannery for preserving fruits and vegetables. In 1934 milk production was 15,378 pounds and butter production at 574 pounds, all from 121 cows. Howard McCoy, Logansport State Hospital dairyman won the 1951 Institutional Dairy Showman Award at the Indiana State Fair. The farm operation at the hospital ceased in 1968. At one time the hospital and its farm covered over thirteen hundred acres.[5, 16-17]

The annual report for the Northern Indiana Hospital for the Insane in 1926 showed a patient population of 1,222 on October 1, 1925. First admissions for psychoses included twelve senile, fourteen arteriosclerotic, thirty-one cerebral syphilis, one Huntington's chorea, eleven manic depressive, six involutional melancholia, sixty dementia praecox, eighteen paranoid, one epileptic, and five with mental deficiency. During 1925 cerebral syphilis was being treated with malaria fever therapy. During that year seventy-seven patients died at the hospital, mostly from senility, cerebral arteriosclerosis, and syphilis.[18]

In 1951 the *Logansport Pharos Tribune* ran a pictorial essay on Logansport State Hospital. This photo essay depicted hypnotherapy, psychosurgery, music therapy, art therapy, psychological testing, and daily staff meetings.[19]

During the 1950s lobotomies were performed at Logansport State Hospital. By the end of 1953 the total number of lobotomies performed stood at 279, a figure which included 232 traditional lobotomies and forty-seven lobotomies using the transorbital technique. Forty-nine (eighteen percent) had been discharged and 193 (sixty-nine percent) had "improved," leaving thirty-seven (thirteen percent) as unimproved. The lobotomy candidates were first screened by three physicians and a psychologist. If accepted for the procedure, the patients were evaluated with a battery of laboratory tests and a battery of psychological tests including the Wechsler Intelligence Scale, Rorschach Ink Blot Test, Draw-a-Person, and Bender Gestalt. The psychological tests were repeated post-surgery. Most of the patients selected for lobotomy were people with chronic schizophrenia with an average duration of illness of eleven years. These patients had failed electroconvulsive therapy and insulin coma therapy. Many were incontinent and/or highly agitated.[20]

Logansport State Hospital's patient population peaked at 2,448 in 1954. During the first seventy-five years of operation the hospital had treated nearly thirty thousand patients.[21-22] In 1959 hospital superintendent Ernest Fogel, M.D., established the hospital's "companion service," in which carefully selected patients became companions and guides for other hospital patients.[23]

In 1993 a new building, which currently houses the majority of patients, was opened. In fiscal year 2009 the average daily population at Logansport State Hospital was 327 and the hospital had 815 employees. Current treatment services include the Dodd Treatment Center, a ninety-six-bed unit for admission and stabilization of adult mental illness patients; the Jayne English Treatment Center, a forty-eight-bed unit for mentally retarded persons; the Southworth West unit with thirty-eight beds for geriatric and medical services; Larson Continuous Psychiatric Services, an eighty-six-bed unit for serious behavioral problems; and the Isaac Ray Treatment Center for forensic patients.[24] One of the more interesting behavioral units in the hospital is for patients with polydipsia or psychogenic water drinking. Currently between eight hundred and one thousand nursing students each year receive training at Logansport State Hospital.

The new Isaac Ray Treatment Center for forensic patients opened in August 2005. The Isaac Ray Treatment Center is a totally separate forensic unit with one hundred five beds housing those found not guilty by reason of insanity, those being made competent to stand trial, and those civil patients having both a serious mental illnesses and dangerous behaviors.[24] About twenty-five percent of the patients housed in the Isaac Ray unit are women.

Logansport State Hospital has a chapel and full-time chaplain on staff. The hospital also has a unique treatment mall, the Fogel Activity Building, which houses a canteen, patient library, beauty and barber shops, bank, and clothing closet where patients can obtain needed clothing. This building also has an auditorium, gymnasium, kitchen, arts and craft room, and game room.[25]

One of the more interesting structures currently on the campus of Logansport State Hospital is the Longcliff Museum, housed in the old pathology building, built in 1911. This museum displays medical and dental instruments, restraint devises, historical photos, news clippings, patient artwork, books, farming equipment, and a television studio. It is well worth a visit as are the remaining beautiful grounds. The stonework at both entrances and the long stone walls were designed by Julius Mattes, a

German immigrant and landscape artist. He began his work in 1892 under superintendent Rogers and continued his work during the administration of Dr. Terflinger.[25-27]

The hospital has two cemeteries. The Old Longcliff Cemetery was abandoned in 1890 and contains no grave markers. The new cemetery lies below the short "cliffs" or rock outcroppings of the hospital grounds along River Road and overlooks the Wabash River. It contains 213 interments. Most of the grave markers are flat and lie embedded in the ground. These markers include names and date of death. There are only two standing gravemarkers.[28] The total number of burials in these two cemeteries is thought to be 561. The first person was buried in 1888 and the last in 1963.[5]

The superintendents of Logansport State Hospital from 1888 to 1967 include the following:

| | |
|---|---|
| Joseph P. Rogers, M.D. | 1888-1908 |
| Fred W. Terflinger, M.D. (Acting) | 1908-1918 |
| Earl Palmer, M.D. | 1918-1919 |
| Fred W. Terflinger, M.D. (Acting) | 1919 |
| Paul E. Bowers, M.D. | 1919-1920 |
| Harvey Elkins, M.D. | 1920 |
| Samuel Dodds, M.D. | 1920-1928 |
| Otis R. Lynch, M.D. | 1928-1933 |
| Clifford L. Williams, M.D. | 1933-1945 |
| Charles C. Chapin, M.D. | 1946-1947 |
| Charles A. Zellers, M.D. | 1948 |
| Richard W. Gohl (Acting) | 1948-1949 |
| John A. Larson, M.D. | 1949-1955 |
| John W. Southworth, M.D. | 1955-1957 |
| Ernest J. Fogel, M.D. | 1958-1967 |

## Richmond State Hospital

The site for the Eastern Indiana Hospital for the Insane, the original name of Richmond State Hospital, was selected in 1878 and occupied slightly over three hundred acres two miles west of Richmond's city center. Construction began in 1884. Initially the first three completed buildings were occupied by the Indiana School for Feeble-Minded Youth, but in 1890 these residents were transferred to what eventually became the Fort Wayne State Developmental Center. Unfortunately most buildings were left in a dilapidated condition, having been unoccupied for several years. The administration building, six cottages, laundry, and boiler house needed extensive renovation. Walls and floors were damaged and defaced. Paint was peeling. The doors did not fit and many had lost their locks. Windows did not work. The sewage and drainage systems were in disrepair as were the roads. The hospital lacked sidewalks. Repair work progressed in record time. In early 1890, the buildings and sewage system were repaired, new water wells were dug, and the hospital grounds were beautified. Despite the neglected state of the farm, a late crop was planted that year and a fair crop of corn, hay, oats and vegetables was harvested. The hospital opened on July 29, 1890 and the first patient was admitted on August 4. By the end of 1890, one hundred and one patients were being treated at the hospital. By mid-1891 there were 303 patients.[1-2]

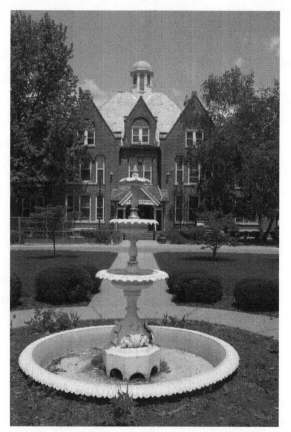

Administration Building, Richmond State Hospital, Richmond, Indiana

In the 1890s daily schedules were signaled by the blast of a steam whistle. Wakeup call was at 5:30 AM in the summer with breakfast served at 6:30. Dinner was at 11:30 AM and supper at 5:30 PM. Lights in patients' rooms were to be out at 9:30 PM.[1]

The hospital was constructed according to a combination of the "cottage plan" (see Dr. Joseph Goodwin Rogers, Chapter 12) and "Kirkbride plans" (see Central State Hospital, Chapter 2). Although never an official name, an early nickname of the hospital was "Easthaven." In the early twentieth century additional farm acreage was purchased so as to allow male inmates with farming experience to work on the lands. The five farms that were acquired were called the "Wayne Farms." This purchase was made possible by a "farm colony law" passed by the Indiana General Assembly in 1911.[3-4]

Until the early 1970s many patients worked on the farms as part of their treatment and rehabilitation. In the early years of hospital-operated farms, the patient workers lived in farm houses which were located on hospital property. These farm houses were named after trees such as Elm House, Maple House, and Pine House. The patients who were farm workers all bunked in one room.

The first fifty-five years of hospital operation highlight changes in American life.[2] In 1892 an outside arc lighting system was installed and a carriage house and ice house were constructed. A railway station was added in 1894 and an "Edison machine," an early phonograph player, was purchased for the entertainment of the patients. By 1898 overcrowding had become a major concern and steps were taken to isolate tuberculous patients in a makeshift hospital. In 1890 three new cottages (Cottage K and Men and Women's Cottages) were built. A new orchard of three hundred apple trees was planted in 1903-04. In 1908 Cottages M and 14 were constructed.

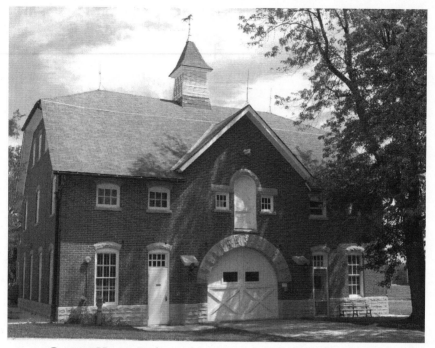

Carriage House, Richmond State Hospital, Richmond, Indiana

In 1909 baths were given to patients only once a week. Women bathed on Mondays and the men on Tuesdays. Bathing hours were either in the mornings or afternoons with each patient bath allotted about ten minutes.[1]

Two patients came down with typhoid in 1913 but both made good recoveries. In the same year a medical building with laboratory, dispensary, and mortuary was constructed and another 446 acres were purchased for Wayne Farms. In 1914 the vineyard produced 15,511 pounds of grapes, and, thanks to the "colony act" of 1911, one hundred and fifty more acres of farmland were purchased. By 1915 there were thirty-two brick buildings and the hospital's capacity was 867. A total of 2,121 bushels of wheat was produced from sixty-four acres. In 1917 another one hundred acres of farmland was purchased. Due to World War I many nurses and attendants left that year to join the military. Mill operations in 1917 produced 119,692 pound of flour and 14,988 pounds of corn meal.

In 1919 a serious fire occurred in the men's cottage and two patients died.[5] Fires have occurred at other Indiana state hospitals, the worst one occurring in 1943 at Evansville State Hospital. After this calamity,

Richmond State Hospital helped out by taking some of their patients, the first arriving on February 10 on the Pennsylvania Railroad.[1]

In the early twentieth century, salaries of hospital personnel were low.[1] In 1909 the superintendent's salary was $333.33 per month. By contrast an assistant physician made one hundred dollars per month. The apothecary or pharmacist was paid fifty dollars per month. In 1905 male supervisors were paid forty-four a month while female supervisors were paid four dollars less. Male day attendants were paid twenty-two dollars a month while female day attendants were paid eighteen dollars. Male night attendants fared better with a monthly salary of thirty-three dollars compared to twenty-one dollars for their female counterparts. The chief cook made fifty dollars per month and the baker was paid forty-five dollars. The head housekeeper's monthly salary was thirty dollars a month and her assistants were paid fourteen dollars. The head farmer was paid sixty dollars a month, a carriage driver thirty dollars, a gardener thirty-five dollars, a teamster twenty dollars, and night watchman thirty-five dollars. All of these employees also received food, lodging, and laundry services. Female attendants dressed in a "blue and white stripped gingham shirt waist and skirt, white linen collar, white apron, and nurse's cap," and their male counterparts dressed in white uniforms.

In 1920 nine patients contracted smallpox and a mass inoculation against this dread disease occurred. In the same year the acreage of Wayne Farms was increased to seven hundred acres by the purchase of 181 more acres of farmland. In 1922 women were moved onto the farm colonies and in 1924 the social service department opened. A new cottage (wards M and N) was constructed. By 1928 bed capacity had grown to 1,171. "Talking pictures," or movies, arrived in 1930. In 1932 a receiving unit for fifty men and fifty women was completed. Hydrotherapy was begun in 1935.

Since the 1930s Richmond State Hospital has had a very active occupational therapy department. In 1951 twenty-one first, second, and third place ribbons were won by hospital patients in the Applied Arts Division at the Indiana State Fair. In addition the hospital has had prize-winning bulls at the State Fair.

Richmond State Hospital was a pioneer in the administration of metrazol and insulin "shock" treatments. Use of these two treatments was begun on July 1, 1938 Although metrazol, a medication that induces seizures, originated in Budapest, Hungary in 1934, it did not appear in the United States until 1938. Initially twenty-two patients with schizophrenia, eleven men and eleven women, were given metrazol intravenously three times a week. By November 1938, of the initial twenty-two patients, four were recovered, four were greatly improved, eight were slightly improved, and six were unimproved. Acutely ill patients improved more than chronic patients. In September 1938, a special building was set aside for the administration of metrazol and insulin "shock" treatments. Insulin coma treatments of schizophrenia originated in Vienna Austria in 1932 and came to the United States in 1936. These treatments were administered by hospital superintendent, Richard Schillinger, M.D., E.F. Jones, M.D., and S.C. Kaim, M.D. Dr. Kaim had previously been in charge of insulin and metrazol treatments at Burg Holzi in Zurich, Switzerland.[6]

In 1939 a new hospital building was completed and in 1940 an auditorium opened. By 1942 bed capacity had grown to 1,701. World War II brought about another acute shortage of personnel. For example in 1945 there were only 188 employees caring for 1,755 patients. By the early 1950s the shortage was so extremely acute because of low pay scales that Richmond State Hospital needed eight physicians for full staffing but had only three and needed thirty-two nurses but had only four. At that time, only South Carolina and Georgia had fewer psychiatric attendants per patient than Indiana.[7] In 1950 the hospital had seventeen hundred patients and the length of stay was seven years. The understaffing was corrected, however in the mid-1950s, and by 1963 the hospital was in good shape again.[8] Between 1952 and 1956 new employee quarters and a new greenhouse were built. In 1961 a new house for the superintendent was constructed and 1970 brought a new chapel.

The annual reports in the early 1950s provide interesting figures. The annual report of the fiscal year ending in June 1954 lists only eight registered nurses on the staff for the entire hospital. During this year there were nearly 120 deaths reported from such causes as stroke (twenty-seven), pneumonia (twenty-one), renal failure (twenty-one), tuberculosis (eleven), and congestive heart failure (ten). The annual report ending in June 1955 indicated that the diet for the previous year relied heavily on dried beans, vegetables, and gravy. Plans for the next year including using less legumes, more sliced meats, surplus foods, a coffee extender, portion control, and leftovers. During that year the hospital baked 184,304 loaves of white bread and 17,291 loaves of rye bread, purchased 8,455 light bulbs, and washed 1,213,075 pounds of laundry. In 1955 the hospital's patients and employees consumed 222,790 pounds of flour.[9-10]

The menus from the 1930s reveal that syrup was often used as a condiment with all three meals. Rolled oats, corn flakes, rice, stewed fruit, frankfurters, or bacon and grits were served at breakfast. The mid-day dinner was the biggest meal of the day, with main dishes of roast pork, beef stew, roast beef, pork and beans, vegetable soup, mutton stew, beef and noodles, and bacon and gravy. Supper, the evening meal, consisted of lighter fare including cheese and crackers, bologna, breaded tomatoes and fruit, navy beans, liver pudding, creamed bologna, southern hash, and navy bean soup.[11-12]

By 1990 the hospital population was down to four hundred patients. In 1991 two new buildings were opened on the Richmond State Hospital campus. One was a 192-bed Residential Treatment Center and the other was a Food Preparation Center. In 2001 a Continued Treatment Center opened and this currently houses laboratory, pharmacy, and dental services as well as classrooms, gym, and crafts area.

Richmond State Hospital is the first state hospital in Indiana to employ "recovery specialists." These former patients have proven especially helpful in insuring adequate treatment and a speedy discharge by imparting a hopeful philosophy to the treatment regimen.

Like other state hospitals, Richmond State Hospital had a cemetery on the hospital grounds for burial of patients whose families could not afford to bury them. The grounds on which the cemetery was located were sold to Wayne County for the county fairgrounds. This cemetery currently has a marker dedicated to the eighty-four patients who are buried there and sits in a grove of trees in the northwest corner of the fairgrounds.

Currently Richmond State Hospital sits on about one hundred acres, has a capacity of three hundred twelve beds, and operates five service lines. The Adult Psychiatric Services consists of a sixty-bed coeducational program for the severely mentally ill. A coeducational Substance Abuse Service has one hundred one beds. The Transitional Service has forty-one coeducational beds and functions to transition the severely mentally ill back into the community. The Life Skills Service is a sixty-bed coeducational service which treats individuals with continuing residual impairments. Finally there is a Specialty Service which houses a thirty-bed coeducational unit for the dually diagnosed (i.e. those individuals with both mental retardation and mental illness).[13] About fifty percent of the patients are voluntary admissions.

The superintendents of Richmond State Hospital from 1890 to 1976 include:

| | |
|---|---|
| Edward F. Wells, M.D. | 1890-1891 |
| Samuel Smith, M.D. | 1891-1923 |
| L.F. Ross, M.D. | 1923-1933 |
| Richard Schillinger, M.D. | 1933-1940 |
| P.S. Johnson, M.D. | 1940-1942 |
| Paul D. Williams, M.D. | 1942-1945 |
| O.R. Lynch, M.D. | 1945-1947 |
| Arthur G. Loftin (Acting) | 1947 |
| Alfred W. Snedeker, M.D. | 1947-1949 |
| L.A. Laird, M.D. | 1949 |
| Paul D. Williams, M.D. | 1949-1953 |
| Arthur G. Loftin (Acting) | 1953 |
| Jefferson Klepfer, M.D. | 1953-1976 |

## Evansville State Hospital

Construction on the Southern Indiana Hospital for the Insane, the first name for what is now Evansville State Hospital, was started in 1888 on one hundred sixty acres of land three miles east of Evansville. The hospital opened for patients on October 30, 1890. Locally the hospital was known as Woodmere, suggesting tranquility in the woods or forest. The original building was massive and built according to the "Kirkbride plan," similar to the Indiana Hospital for the Insane in Indianapolis. A fence was built around the hospital and landscaping, including trees, fountains, and paths, were added. Beginning in 1895 and extending to 1927, four additional wings were added to the original hospital. A separate building, the "sick hospital" was added in 1911. This hospital, which treated the medical illnesses of mentally ill patients, contained an operating room, laboratory, tuberculosis ward, and morgue. Other buildings included a carpenter shop, well house, railway station, greenhouse, assembly hall, bakery, laundry, dairy and stock barns, carriage house, and two silos. An employees' building, containing ninety-eight single rooms and two apartments, was completed in 1941.[1-3]

Not long after the hospital had opened, superintendent Andrew Thomas, M.D., and his assistant Dr. Waring took some of the *Evansville Journal's* staff on a tour of the magnificent new facility. The *Journal's* staff seemed duly impressed:

"The administration building is entered from the portico into the reception area…the visitor steps into an entry hall, with decorated walls, polished floors, and comfortably cushioned divans…On the left is the private office of Dr. Thomas…fitted up with desk and chairs of elegant pattern…On the right comes first the record room and telephone exchange…The two upper stories of the administration building are occupied…[on] the second by Dr. Thomas…while the third floor is occupied by the assistant physicians…Leaving the administration building you pass through the "arcade" to the asylum proper… the central block [of the] building is in the shape of a six-pointed star, and from this central hub everyone of the twelve wards radiate…"[4]

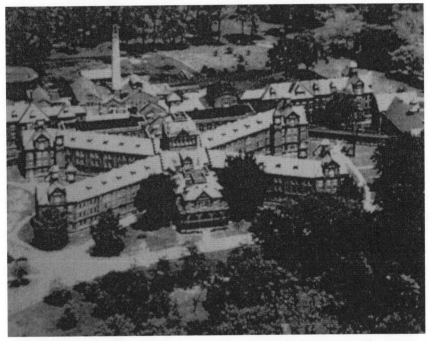

Main Building, Evansville State Hospital, Evansville, Indiana, early 1900s

The *Journal's* staff viewed the train arrival of fifty patients from the Central Indiana Hospital for the Insane in Indianapolis:

"When word was given to the superintendent that 'the train is here' he had his attendants marshaled and prepared for the work at hand...there was a large crowd of people waiting to see the unfortunates debark...As the patients came down from the cars, led by a blue-coated Indianapolis official...There was one young man in the crowd who believes that God and Edison together created the world, and that he now controls them both. He kept up a constant talking that seemed to amuse the onlookers very much..."[4]

When the hospital first opened, Superintendent Thomas asked each county clerk in the hospital's district to send two individuals from each of that county's poor houses and jails, excluding those with epilepsy and severe medical illnesses.[5] Initially all patients were required to wear uniforms, consisting of pajamas, hospital gown and soft shoes, in order to make escape more difficult. Within the first year of hospital operation Superintendent Thomas had the employees organize an orchestra. He also organized a leisure reading program.[3]

By the early 1940s Evansville State Hospital was a bustling city within a city. The hospital grounds consisted of eight hundred eighty acres, five hundred of which were cultivated. The hospital farm produced fruit, vegetables, cattle, hogs, and chickens. At one time it contained as many as one hundred cows, five hundred pigs, and five thousand chickens. Beans, pumpkins, potatoes, turnips, tomatoes, and cucumbers were among the hospital's vegetable produce. The hospital grounds housed laboratory and dental offices, barber and beauty shops, an industrial shop, a canteen, and farm buildings including a dairy. Patients were employed in various occupations in the hospital and upon the grounds, including farming, sewing, laundry, housekeeping, and kitchen work.[3]

Evansville State Hospital enjoyed many unique programs. It was the second psychiatric hospital in the United States to have a Gavel Club, an affiliate of Toastmaster's International. It was the first psychiatric hospital to have a Homemaker's Club.[3]

Over the years Evansville State Hospital offered a number of somatic therapies including hydrotherapy, metrazol convulsive therapy, insulin coma therapy, electroconvulsive therapy, lobotomies, and atropine coma therapy. The last lobotomy was performed at the hospital in 1960.[3]

Like other Indiana state psychiatric hospitals, Evansville State Hospital has had crises. The first occurred at 2:30 AM on February 9, 1943 when a fire erupted in the main building at the hospital. The building was three stories tall and included administrative offices, the dining hall, and four dormitory wings for patients. At the time of the fire, this building contained one half of the total hospital space with 1,180 patients housed in its dormitories.

Within minutes of the fire being discovered, John H. Hare, M.D., hospital superintendent, was awakened from his quarters in the building. Dr. Hare led a heroic effort in arousing other staff, unlocking the dormitories, and evacuating the patients. He led these efforts in the chilly night-time air while shirtless and wearing a worn leather jacket. Initially patients were led to the hospital grounds. Restraining ward patients were placed in the theater and greenhouses. Most of the patients remained calm and orderly. One female patient, however, became agitated and threw flower pots at policemen in the greenhouse when they tried to calm her.

Within minutes, Evansville firemen responded and by the time the fire was extinguished, seven fire companies and all auxiliary fire companies were involved. Seventy-five members of Company G of the Indiana Guard responded as did state and city police.

During the fire a few patients wandered from the hospital grounds. A day after the fire about twenty patients were still missing. One patient was finally located in Illinois.

On the night of the fire only one person, an employee, Ida McIntire, linen maker, was thought to have perished in the fire. Another employee, Maud Maxwell, supervisor of women, was missing. Years later the *Evansville Courier* reported that six patients and two employees, Ms McIntire and Ms Maxwell, had died in the fire. The reports of the number of those who perished in the fire remains uncertain.

Later on the same day of the fire, plans were formulated by Governor Henry Schricker and Dr. Hare to transfer the patients to other state facilities. A Chicago and Eastern Illinois train, including thirteen coaches and four baggage cars, was assembled at Terre Haute and sent to Evansville. Three hundred patients were to be sent by train to Logansport State Hospital and seven hundred to Central State Hospital. One hundred patients were taken to Madison State Hospital by bus. Other Indiana facilities accepting patients included the Indiana Girls School in Claremont, the Muscatatuck State Colony, and the Indiana Village for the Insane in New Castle.[7]

Since most records were destroyed, a number of patients arrived at these other state institutions without records of their names. Some did not know their names and a few concocted fictitious names. Some denied they had been patients.

Fortunately, the Indiana State Legislature was in session when the fire occurred. On the day after the fire legislative leaders from the State Budget Committee and the House Ways and Means Committee sprung into action. Soon plans were made to ask permission from the War Production Board to procure materials and begin construction of a new hospital.[8]

Construction on a new administration building was started in the spring of 1943. In September 1943 the G.K. Newberry Construction Company of Chicago cleared debris from the burned out building. The architects of the new building were McGuire and Shook of Indianapolis. The new building housing patients was to consist of 350,000 square feet and was budgeted to cost two million dollars. Construction was completed by 1945.[9]

On June 25, 1945 the *Indianapolis News* reported that forty-one male patients were transferred from Logansport State Hospital back to Evansville State Hospital in Army jeeps. In the same manner thirty-five female patients had been transferred the day before.

Another low point for Evansville State Hospital occurred in November 1968 when hospital superintendent Milton H. Anderson, M.D., was fired. His firing caused five of the six remaining physicians on the staff to resign.[10-11]

In the late 1960s and early 1970s Evansville State Hospital faced another crisis when massive budget cuts were imposed by the Indiana State Legislature. The hospital's rehabilitation programs suffered the greatest, since nurses were retained at the expense of rehabilitation personnel. The fiscal crisis was so great that in 1973 Superintendent Ernest Fogel, M.D., halted admissions.[3]

Beginning in 1958 a number of new buildings were added to Evansville State Hospital. These included an activity therapy building with canteen, gymnasium, and auditorium. In the summer of 1964 a split level building for one hundred fifty patients, mostly geriatric, was opened. That year the patient population was 1,150 housed on thirty-seven wards. Seven physicians including three psychiatrists were on the staff, along with thirty-one nurses, ten social workers and four psychologists. Of the total of five hundred employees, 259 were attendants.[12]

Most of the original land for the hospital has been sold, so currently only about two hundred acres remain. St. Mary's Medical Center purchased eighty acres in 1951 and in 1959 Indiana transferred five hundred acres to the Indiana Department of Conservation. In 1967 the University of Evansville bought forty acres. In 1988 the Southwestern Indiana Mental Health Center was built on the grounds.[1-3]

By the end of the 1974-75 fiscal year the number of beds at Evansville State Hospital was down to 871 with 440 beds for men and 431 for women. During that year there were 454 full and part-time employees.[5] By the end of 2008 all of the old buildings at Evansville State Hospital had been demolished. In September 2003 a new 168-bed hospital opened. The current hospital is composed of three services: the developmental training services with thirty-two beds, the medical/geriatric service with thirty-four beds, and the admissions/adult continuing treatment service with 102 beds. The hospital has a centralized "treatment mall," containing classrooms, teaching kitchen, library, music room, computer lab, hair salon, and arts and crafts area. This new hospital is connected by a covered connector to a newly renovated activity building which contains a gymnasium, bowling alley, and canteen.[13-14]

As at other state hospitals, indigent patients whose families could not afford burial were buried on the hospital grounds. The exact sites and numbers of patients buried on the grounds of Evansville State Hospital are unknown. However, in 1984 during the construction of the Lloyd Expressway thirty-six graves were discovered and the remains were re-interred at Evansville's Memorial Park Cemetery. Another thirty-three graves were discovered in 1987 and moved to Memorial Park Cemetery.[15]

In 1990 a number of twenty-plus year employees offered their memories for the one hundredth year anniversary of the hospital.[3]

> "[We] were required to wear a white, starched uniform and polished shoes. Once each month we had an eleven day stretch to work before getting our three day weekend off...Nothing would quiet an agitated patient quicker than the old 'ice pack'..."

Floyd Greulich, psychiatric attendant

> "...my first day of employment...I came to work in street clothes...They assigned me to the men's hospital ward...I spent my first day feeding and bathing patients...A little

after 3 p.m...I noticed that the guys I was working with were gone...I had not been issued ward keys...I asked one of the second shift guys to unlock the door...[he said] 'go into the day room and sit down...don't cause any trouble'...I told him to call my supervisor...[but] he had left for the day and also that the second shift supervisor had never heard of me...now I was getting worried...[but] Miss Thomas, the Director of Nursing remembered me and they finally let me off the ward..."

William Mauer, Housekeeping Director

"Dr. Anderson was our psychiatrist and superintendent. He would walk through the wards every day...The nurses would call ahead and say "Andy" is on his way...We would all see everything was in order. He did not want to see a wrinkle on a bed..."

Gloria Paul, Psychiatric Attendant

"When I first came to the state hospital over 30 years ago...We shaved all male patients three times a week and gave them a haircut once a month."

Dale M. Melton

"One patient I will always remember. When I would get finished with his teeth he would pull out a piece of toilet paper from his pocket and write me a check for a million dollars!"

Robert L. Miley, D.D.S.

The superintendents of Evansville State Hospital from 1890 to 1981 include the following:

| | |
|---|---|
| Andrew J. Thomas, M.D. | 1890-1897 |
| George C. Mason, M.D. | 1897-1900 |
| William A. Stoker | 1900-1903 |
| Charles E. Loughlin, M.D. | 1903-1933 |
| John H. Hare, M.D. | 1933-1952 |
| H.M. Kauffman, M.D. | 1952-1953 |

| | |
|---|---|
| Milton H. Anderson, M.D. | 1953-1969 |
| H.S. Gillespie, M.D. (Acting) | 1969 |
| Joseph H. McCool, M.D. | 1969-1972 |
| Ernest F. Fogel, M.D. | 1972-1976 |
| Spiro Mitsos, M.D. | 1976-1981 |

## CHAPTER 4

# Twentieth Century Public Psychiatric Hospitals in Indiana

This yet unnamed new hospital, later to be known as Larue D. Carter Memorial Hospital was "to be made available for instruction of medical students, student nurses, interns and resident physicians under the supervision of the faculty of the Indiana University School of Medicine for use by said school in connection with research and instruction in psychiatric disorders."

> An act concerning mental cases, creating the Indiana Council for Mental Health and prescribing its powers and duties, authorizing the construction of a hospital, providing for admission thereto and release therefrom and making an appropriation, and providing for enforcement. *Laws of the state of Indiana, Regular session of the 84*[th] *Indiana General Assembly*. Indianapolis, Indiana: Bookwalter Company, 1945, pp. 1571.

## Madison State Hospital[1]

Madison State Hospital, located on a four hundred foot bluff, known affectionately as "the Hill," overlooks Madison, Indiana and the Ohio River. The hospital likely has the most picturesque location of all of the state psychiatric hospitals in the United States. It is adjacent to and just east of Clifty Falls State Park. Sadly, it is much smaller in recent years due to much of the beautiful grounds being taken over by the Madison Correctional Facility, a minimum security prison established in 1989 for female inmates, who are housed in many of the hospital's former patient cottages. Fences topped with razor wire surround the Madison Correctional Facility. Many of the campus's beautiful trees had to be cut to accommodate the land's new use. A "catwalk" or stairs connects with the Heritage Trail of Madison, which comes up from below the bluff.

The construction of Madison State Hospital was authorized by the Indiana State Legislature in 1905 in order to relieve the overcrowding in the three other state psychiatric hospitals. Originally 363 acres were purchased for $39,214.84. The "cottage" concept was adapted as a design, a radical departure from the massive buildings housing psychiatric patients at the turn of the twentieth century. The original hospital construction included twenty-two two-story buildings which could accommodate thirty wards with twenty to seventy beds apiece. Other original buildings included an administration building, a service building with kitchen and dining rooms, powerhouse, laundry, workshop, and an industrial building. The campus was divided into male and female sides. Patients from each side ate and recreated at different times of the day and week. The original cost of Madison State Hospital was $1,172,217.30.[2-3]

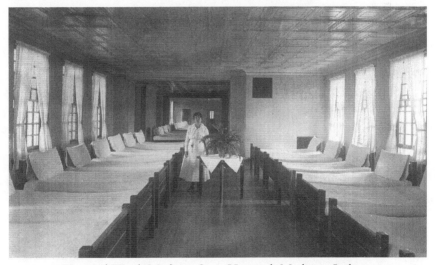

Hospital Ward, Madison State Hospital, Madison, Indiana

A pumping station pumped water from the Ohio River for storage in a large water tower. The powerhouse was fueled by coal but was abandoned in 1950 when the campus was converted from DC current and purchased local AC current.

Originally called the Southeastern Indiana Hospital for the Insane, the hospital began accepting its first 476 southeastern Indiana patients from Central State Hospital in Indianapolis in August 1910. Patients were brought by train and were escorted by guards toting shotguns loaded with rock salt. By the end of 1910 there were 544 patients and seventy-four employees. By 1915 there were about one thousand patients and by the 1930s, 110 attendants were caring for 1,585 patients. To ease overcrowding, four nearby farm homes were purchased for the men and a cottage was built for eighty women. Originally constructed for 1,250 patients, Madison State Hospital at one time housed about eighteen hundred patients. Known locally as "Cragmont," the hospital's name was changed to Madison State Hospital in 1927.

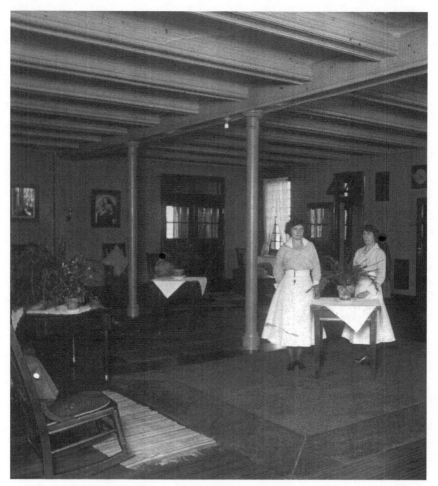

Women's Ward Day Room, Madison State Hospital, Madison, Indiana

From its early days Madison State Hospital, like some of the other Indiana state psychiatric hospitals, was a farming colony. At one time the hospital grounds consisted of 1265 acres, with five hundred acres devoted to farming. Its produce, including apples, plums, peaches, grapes, green beans, cabbage, sweet corn, wheat, potatoes, eggs, beef, pork, eggs, chickens, geese, and turkey, was used to feed the patients and employees. The farm was so successful, that between 1916 and 1938, Madison State Hospital returned $225,000 in profit to the Indiana state treasury...and this was in the middle of the Great Depression. Originally attendants worked twelve-hour days seven days a week, but in 1950 an eight-hour workday was established with a forty-eight hour work week.

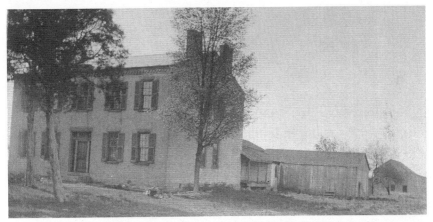

Colony II Farmhouse, Madison State Hospital, Madison, Indiana

Early therapies included hydrotherapy, cold packs, and showers. In the late 1920s malarial therapy was introduced for the treatment of general paresis and in the late 1930s insulin and metrazol shock therapies began to be utilized. Early research efforts included the study of Huntington's disease and criminal sexual psychopaths. In 1953 a Saturday outpatient clinic was established. In the late 1960s developmentally disabled patients began treatment at Madison State Hospital. The 1970s saw the establishment of treatment for drug and alcohol addiction and adolescent patients.

Madison State Hospital has had its ups and downs. It was first accredited by the Joint Commission on Hospital Accreditation Organization (JCAHO) in 1962, but lost its accreditation in 1971 because of lack of a sprinkler system. It passed its most recent JCAHO accreditation in 2007 with flying colors. It is Medicare and Medicaid certified. During World War I, the Great Depression, and World War II, staffing levels were greatly reduced. For example, during World War II, two physicians and ninety-six attendants cared for seventeen hundred patients. The daily cost to run the hospital was $3.72 per patient in 1911, but this was decreased to $.475 in 1934. By the 1983-84 year the daily cost per patient was $81.00 for 429 patients. The 1918 influenza epidemic caused a few deaths. The April 1974 tornado destroyed half of the trees on the campus and caused over a million dollars damage. Fortunately no lives were lost.

Although the beautiful two-story administration building remains, two patient-care buildings (buildings thirteen and twenty-one) were torn down, reconstructed, and connected to building two, consisting of A, B, and C wings, housing an auditorium, gym, patient library, barber/beauty shop, library, conference rooms, and medical and dental clinics.[4]

The new buildings were designed by the St. Louis-based HOK and the Indianapolis-based Ratio architectural firms. The buildings have earned the LEED (Leadership in Energy and Environmental Design) certification from the US Green Building Council.[5] These new air-conditioned buildings are energy-efficient and allow for maximum daylighting through the use of skylights, clerestories, and highly fenestrated hallways. Recycling is encouraged through the through installation of recycling containers. A unique feature is an electronic identification badge, which allows patients access and egress to parts of the buildings and grounds based upon their privilege level.

Since 2003, Peggy Stephens, MD, has been superintendent and medical director. Dr. Stephens is triple-boarded (general, addictions, & geriatric psychiatry) and is a distinguished fellow of the American Psychiatric Association. She is a past president of the Kentucky Psychiatric Society.[6]

During fiscal year 2008 the average daily population at Madison State Hospital was 133.2 patients and there were 467 full time staff working there. The hospital is currently configured for ninety adult psychiatric patients and sixty patients with mental retardation and/or developmental disabilities.[7] Currently Madison State Hospital contains six adult units, four units for patients with mental retardation and/or developmental disabilities units, and an eighteen-bed geriatric unit. Some units are coed. The hospital utilizes a team-treatment approach with seven-day-a-week programming. Madison State Hospital offers patient and family educational groups, activity-related groups, psychotherapy groups, and transitional groups. The campus is entirely smoke-free, a first for any Indiana state psychiatric hospital. The staff currently includes five treating psychiatrists. Hospital clinics include internal medicine, dental, ophthalmology, and podiatry clinics. Radiology services are provided by King's Daughters Hospital in Madison. Blood work is sent to outside laboratories with results available by computer. Some clinicians are dually trained. For example, a recreational therapist also does music therapy and the hospital chaplain does art therapy. Sadly, the hospital's museum, which housed many interesting articles and pictures, was closed about a year ago.

Currently all patients are involuntary. The hospital houses patients who have been judged incompetent to stand trial and those who have been found not guilty by reason of insanity. The former patients participate in legal education designed to restore them to competency. Medication orders are sent to the pharmacy via computer. The hospital staff is striving to decrease polypharmacy and have instituted a twice-daily dosing system to simplify medication use for transition and discharge. Eventually all medical records will be computerized.

Another unique treatment feature at Madison State Hospital is the Record of Daily Functioning and Treatment Progress (DPT). A daily DPT form is maintained on all patients. This form contains areas for activities of daily living, symptoms, and various treatments. Information is hand-entered. Night shift ward personnel transcribe this information to a "daily total/weekly averages worksheet." The "safety seven" items enumerated include physical aggression, verbal threats, sexual aggression, self-injury, property destruction, elopement, and other safety measures. From these records a seven-page "Record of Monthly Summary" is generated. This record contains summaries from the attending physician, nursing, social service, and rehabilitation therapies. It is used for both patient and family education and is an indispensable treatment tool. None of the other state psychiatric hospitals currently have this tool. It has allowed Madison State Hospital to minimize the use of as needed medications and seclusion and restraint. A final unique feature is a report, which is periodically sent to the Indiana Division of Mental Health and the community mental health centers which follow patients discharged from Madison State Hospital.

In summary, Madison State Hospital has a fascinating history and is currently a leader in care for Indiana's disadvantaged adult psychiatric and mentally retarded/developmentally disabled patient populations.

The superintendents of Madison State Hospital from 1910 to 1979 are:

| | |
|---|---|
| Edward P. Busse, M.D. | 1910-1915 |
| James W. Milligan, M.D. | 1915-1944 |

| John H. Hare, M.D. | 1944 |
| L.E. Pennington, M.D. | 1944-1945 |
| George W. Bander, M.D. | 1945-1947 |
| Charles A. Zitter, M.D. | 1947-1948 |
| M.W. Kemp, M.D. | 1948-1952 |
| Ott B. McAtee, M.D. | 1952-1979 |

## Larue D. Carter Memorial Hospital

The building of Larue D. Carter Memorial Hospital was authorized by the Indiana General Assembly in 1945.[1] However, due to budgetary concerns, construction did not begin until January 10, 1948 when ground was officially broken. The initial estimated cost of Carter Hospital was $2,187,000, but by 1951 its cost had ballooned to five million dollars. The first patient was admitted to Carter in July 1952 although the construction was not complete until 1953. Located on the campus of Indiana University Medical Center, Carter Hospital was envisioned as a training ground for psychiatrists, social workers, psychologists, nurses, occupational therapists, and medical students.[2-6]

The building, designed by Frost, Daggett, and Associates in Indianapolis, was constructed in six different units connected by joints which allowed for expansion and contraction of its concrete. The V-shaped wings located at each end of the building were designed to allow for the segregation of male and female patients. The floors of the central section of the building housed laboratories, offices, kitchens, dining rooms, and auditorium. The T-shaped front of the building housed reception areas on three floors, administrative offices, conference rooms, class rooms. The second and third floors originally housed offices for the Indiana Mental Health Council, forerunner to the Department of Mental Health. The fourth floor of this wing contained the residence of the hospital superintendent. Initially walls were painted pastel tints of green, gray, tan, coral, and blue. The asphalt floor tiles were tan, gray, red, and green. The walls of the hospital wards were glazed block and the floors were terrazzo. Much of the hospital furnishings were crafted at the Indiana State Prison. Patient rooms were furnished with beds, chairs, and clothes closets and each ward had its own living room area and screened-in porch. The hospital contained a patient library, snack bar, beauty and barber shop, occupational and recreational therapy departments, and a well-stocked professional library. The occupational therapy department was equipped with looms, jewelry and basket making equipment, leather making and woodworking equipment, painting supplies, and facilities to make ceramics. Initially food was brought in from a central commissary which served all of the Indiana University Medical Center hospitals. The food arrived at Carter Hospital's four finishing kitchens through a series of tunnels connecting the hospital with the medical center. The basement of Carter Hospital's northeast wing, which housed the outpatient department, had its own outside entrance and reception area. Initially offices for psychologists and social workers were housed in the outpatient department.[7]

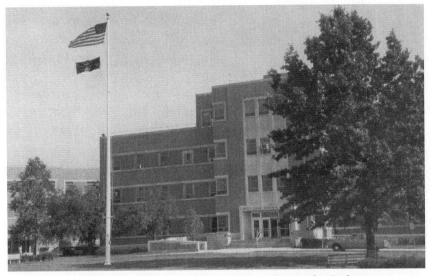

Larue D. Carter Memorial Hospital, Indianapolis, Indiana

The hospital was officially dedicated on September 28, 1952. It was named for Larue D. Carter, M.D., the first president of the Indiana Council for Mental Health. Dr. Carter had been a professor of neuropsychiatry at Indiana University School of Medicine, chief of psychiatry at Indianapolis City Hospital, and medical director of Norways Sanitarium, a private psychiatric hospital in Indianapolis. Initially admission to Carter Hospital was by one of two procedures, either by voluntary application or by a temporary ninety-day commitment through the circuit court systems of Indiana's counties.[8]

The staffing of Carter Hospital got off to a slow start because of low pay scales. Employee recruitment began in December 1951 under the direction of Juul C. Nielsen, M.D., the hospital's newly appointed superintendent. The first patients were admitted on July 26, 1952. At that time in Indiana the monthly pay ranges were $700-845 a month for hospital superintendents, $600-745 for psychiatric physicians, $225-345 for psychiatry residents, and $200-320 for psychiatric nurses. The hospital's initial bed capacity was to be two hundred fifty patients with one hundred beds for women, one hundred for men, and fifty for children.[9]

By November 1952 the hospital only had filled forty-six beds. Indianapolis Mayor Alex Clark criticized the hospital for not relieving the overcrowding of mental patients at the Marion County Jail and General Hospital. He even went so far as to instruct Gerald Kempf, M.D., superintendent of General Hospital, to send its psychiatric patients and those admitted under a pre-mental examination writ directly to Carter Hospital, but Carter's superintendent, Dr. Nielsen, responded that they did not have enough qualified staff to treat them because of low pay scales.[10-11]

By June 1953 Carter Hospital had filled only ninety-two beds because pay scales still had not been increased by the state. The children's ward still had not been opened. The Marion County Jail had contained twenty-two adult patients awaiting psychiatric examination.[12] In July 1953 an idea was floated by Indianapolis Mayor Clark that Indianapolis lease space at Carter Hospital for psychiatric patients housed in the city jail, but apparently this idea never came to fruition.[13] By August 1953 the Indiana mental health commissioner, Margaret Morgan, M.D., announced that Carter Hospital would increase bed capacity to 150 by opening hospital beds to relieve overcrowding at General Hospital, freeing General Hospital to reduce overcrowding at the Marion County Jail. By October 1, Dr. Morgan had planned to have two hundred adult patients and by January of 1954 have fifty additional beds open for children. This increase in patient population was made possible by an increase in the salary scale by the state budget agency.[14]

The children's unit at Carter Hospital finally opened in October, 1954 on the hospital's third floor. This unit, for children ages six to twelve, was to contain twenty-five beds. This unit's opening was delayed because its new director, William L. Lordi, M.D., was stricken with polio during the summer of 1954. This new unit was finally able to take the pressure off other Indiana state mental hospitals which had been hospitalizing children an adult wards. One of the first children admitted to the children's ward was an eleven-year boy who had been hospitalized on an adult men's ward at Central State Hospital.[15-16]

During the 1954-55 fiscal year, Carter Hospital had five psychiatrists: Juul Nielsen, M.D, superintendent, Edward Hinko, M.D., assistant superintendent, August Yochen, M.D., clinical director, Anthony Polock, M.D., chief of the outpatient department, and Margaret Hatfield, M.D., chief of the Alcohol Service. Junior medical students began rotating through the hospital in groups of fifteen and spent five afternoons a week at Carter. During that year 3,951 insulin coma treatments were given to fifty-six women and forty-eight men. Seventy-seven men and 149 women had a collective total of 3,987 electroconvulsive treatments, an average of about eighteen treatments per patient. Of the three patient deaths that occurred that year, two occurred while patients were on leaves of absence. One hundred and sixty-two alcoholics were admitted and ninety-seven patients were treated in the outpatient department.[17]

Dr. Nielsen resigned as superintendent of Carter Hospital in May 1955. Unfortunately Dr. Nielsen's resignation was shortly followed by the resignations of five other Carter Hospital psychiatrists and nine residents, leaving only two psychiatrists and six residents to run the entire hospital. Three social work supervisors left that year, so the training of social workers was suspended. The mass exodus of personnel was thought to be at least partially caused by not having a full-time chair of Department of Psychiatry for the previous two years.[18]

Fortunately a rescuer was about to arrive to take over as superintendent of Carter Hospital. Donald F. Moore, M.D., arrived on October 1. He was immediately saddled with the enormous job of recruiting psychiatrists, which was made even harder by the continuing problem of a low salary scale for state hospital psychiatrists.

By 1955 Thorazine, psychiatry's new wonder drug, had arrived at Carter Hospital. Thorazine, along with reserpine, which had been in use for three years at Carter, was being used to treat agitation in schizophrenia. At the time, Thorazine was so new that its side effects were not completely known. Meprobamate was being used to calm anxiety in less severe clinical conditions.[19]

In September 1955 Marion DeMyer, M.D. took over head of the children's ward at Carter Hospital. Dr. DeMyer and her colleagues initiated a seven-year research program to study childhood schizophrenia and childhood autism and their small group eventually published a number of pioneering professional papers and books on autism.[20]

In 1965 psychiatrists Drs. Joyce and Iver Small were recruited to begin an aggressive clinical research program. Over the succeeding years the

Research Service conducted groundbreaking research on the use of lithium carbonate in bipolar disorder, electroconvulsive therapy, and research on many of the newer second and third generation antipsychotic medications, including clozapine.

Beginning in 1968 a small revolution began at Carter Hospital with the gradual unlocking of the doors to patient wards. Doors were unlocked on the adult units with the exception of the admission and research wards. The onerous need to write passes for patients and have nursing staff continue locking and unlocking ward doors was finally over.[21-22]

On July 1, 1974 the Psychology Department received a $200,000 grant for a three-year follow-up study of the hospital's patients. Paul Martin, Ph.D., the project's principal investigator, and Arthur Sterne, Ph.D., the chief of the Psychology Department were heavily involved in this project over the next several years. This project had been preceded by a pilot follow-up project beginning in 1971. One early finding of the study was that patients complained about gaining weight on hospital food and this resulted in dietary modifications. An interesting later finding was that therapists' expectancies for therapeutic gain were positively associated with treatment outcome. This project ultimately resulted in the publication in professional psychology journals of a score of articles on this study.[23-24]

In the 1979-80 fiscal year at Carter Hospital 421 patients were admitted to the hospital and 603 new patients were seen in the outpatient department. Most patients (316) were admitted by voluntary application. The readmission rate was about eighteen percent. The distribution of diagnoses on the adult, children and adolescent services was: schizophrenia (one hundred fourteen), personality disorders (fifty-five), affective disorders (thirty-seven), organic brain syndromes (twenty-six), behavior disorders (twenty-four), other psychoses (seventeen), transient situational disturbances (sixteen), other neuroses (fourteen), and other disorders (sixteen) for a total of 319 patients. The average length of stay, excluding leaves of absence, was eighty-nine days on the Adult Service, 140 days on the Adolescent Service, and 145 days on the Children's Service. The Carter Hospital training programs educated twenty-seven psychiatric residents, four neurology residents, six psychology interns, 596 medical students, eleven social workers, nine clergy chaplains, eight special education teachers, eighty-seven nursing students, eighteen occupational therapy students, two recreational therapy students, three music therapy students, and one medical records student that year. By 1981 the hospital had trained 244 psychiatric and neurologic physicians of whom 158 were known to be practicing in Indiana and seventy-one out of state. Of the psychiatrists trained, 103 had entered private practice and sixty-six were working in other public psychiatric facilities including community mental health centers.[22] During the 1982-1983 year Carter Hospital admitted 313 adults and sixty-nine children and adolescents while the Outpatient Department admitted 275 patients.[25]

In 1996 Carter Hospital was moved from its original location at 1315 West 10th Street to a new location at 2601 Cold Springs Road in Indianapolis where it took over the spacious grounds of the former Cold Springs Road Veterans Administration Hospital. Currently the hospital has 159 beds. These beds are spread over a number of wards including two general adult wards, a ward treating patients with borderline personality disorder, a research unit, a unit for deaf patients, and child and adolescent units.

Superintendents of Carter Hospital from 1951 through 1989 include:

| | |
|---|---|
| Juul C. Nielsen. M.D. | 1951-1955 |
| Edward N. Hinko, M.D. (Acting) | 1955 |
| Margaret Morgan, M.D. (Acting) | 1955 |
| Donald Moore, M.D. | 1955-1980 |
| Clare Assue, M.D. | 1980-1989 |

CHAPTER 5

# Private Psychiatric Institutions

## NEURONHURST

Dr. W.B. Fletcher's Sanitorium for Nervous and Mental Diseases
A strictly psychopathic hospital for the treatment of all forms of
Neuropsychoses by proper medication, careful nursing, and general
hygienic treatment, in conjunction with the most modern and
approved electric and hydrotherapeutic measures.
Baths and Massage
Facilities for Turkish, Nauheim, and other baths
For terms and further particulars address
Dr. Mary A. Spink, Superintendent
Phone, Riley 3636
1140 E. market Street, Indianapolis, Ind.

Advertisement for Neuronhurst
in the *Indianapolis Directory*, 1937

This chapter is not intended to give an extensive review of private psychiatric hospitals and hospital units in Indiana. In fact, only three will be discussed: the Fletcher Sanitarium or Neuronhurst, Norways Hospital, and the psychiatric wing at Methodist Hospital in Indianapolis. Beginning in the 1950s many private not-for-profit hospitals in Indiana established psychiatric units and beginning in the 1970s many for-profit psychiatric hospitals, such as the Charter Hospital chain, proliferated.

## Neuronhurst[1-4]

In 1888 Dr. William Fletcher opened the Fletcher Sanitorium, later known as Neuronhurst, the first private facility for the treatment of nervous and mental diseases in Indiana. He immediately hired Mary Angela Spink,

M.D., as his assistant. Neuronhurst had at least three different locations, one on North Alabama Street, another at Pennsylvania Avenue and North Street, and the third at Market Street and Highland Avenue. Eventually the institution had a capacity of fifty beds. Both voluntary and committed patients were accepted for treatment. A gymnasium and swimming pool were available for exercise. Close personal supervision was provided with a minimum of restraint. Diets were carefully prepared in kitchens and numerous types of therapeutic baths were provided including saline, Turkish, steam, light ray, and ozone. A well-equipped laboratory was on site. When not engaged in therapies, patients could enjoy the gardens and solarium.

The 1930 United States census for the "W.B. Fletcher Sanitarium (Insane)" listed sixteen employees, including three physicians and eight nurses, and thirteen patients, including nine females and four males, who ranged in age from twenty-six to ninety-seven years.

When Dr. Fletcher died in 1907, Dr. Mary Spink took over as director. She was assisted by her sister, Urbana Spink, M.D., a graduate of the Woman's Medical College in Philadelphia. Both Dr. Fletcher and Dr. Spink were extraordinary neuropsychiatrists. Dr. Fletcher was an innovator and far ahead of his times. Dr. Spink was highly accomplished and pioneered the way for women in Indiana medicine. Neuronhurst closed shortly after the death of Dr. Spink in 1937.

## Norways Hospital[1]

If you were a resident in the Department of Psychiatry at Indiana University School of Medicine in Indianapolis, Indiana, you are no doubt familiar with the picture of Norways Hospital which used to hang in the library at the Institute of Psychiatric Research.

Established in 1898, Norways Hospital was the second private psychiatric hospital established in Indianapolis. Norways Hospital, originally known as Norways Sanitarium, was founded by Albert E. Sterne, M.D., the first professor of nervous and mental disease at Indiana University School of Medicine. The hospital became known as Norways Foundation Hospital in 1943. The hospital was named Norways because of the many Norway maple trees growing on the two-acre estate of Stoughton A. Fletcher and family, whose residence, built in 1870, served as the first hospital building. In the first ten years of Norways' existence, two new buildings were added. A final building was completed in 1946. At its founding, there were ten beds and this number was doubled in the second year. By the hospital's closing in 1957, it contained sixty-nine beds. The hospital was located on Indianapolis' near east side at 1820 East 10th Street.[2-5]

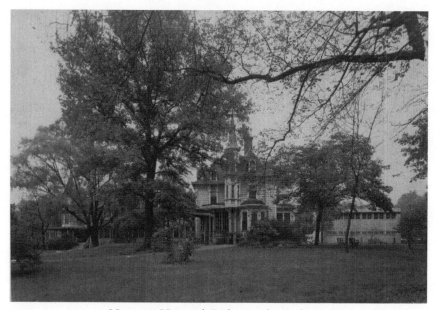

Norways Hospital, Indianapolis, Indiana

One of Dr. Sterne's lesser-known accomplishments was a technique, presumably developed while he was at Norways, for the treatment of neurasthenia. Subsequently Dr. Sterne published, "Neurasthenia and its treatment by actinic rays," in the *Journal of the American Medical Association*. For this particular treatment Dr. Sterne had a cabinet constructed in which the neurasthenic patient sat unclothed and whose body was bathed with "primeval actinic rays" produced by arc lamps and vacuum tubes while his or her head was bathed in air charged with ozone. This treatment was said to decrease the time of treatment of a neurasthenic patient by half.[6]

Albert Sterne, M.D., of course, was the first medical director of Norways Hospital. Philip Reed, M.D., was medical director at Norways for about twenty years until it closed in 1957. His wife, Genevieve, was the executive director.

Norways Hospital always had state-of-the-art treatment. X-ray fluoroscopy was introduced in 1899. Brain surgery was performed there as early as 1910. Insulin coma therapy was introduced in 1937 and new techniques for its administration were developed at Norways. In 1938 the use of Metrazol shock was introduced and electroconvulsive therapy was begun in 1940.[3] Patients with mania were treated with paraldehyde and wet sheet packs. Still later, occupational therapy and music therapy were introduced. In the early 1950s Dr. Robert Bill, for many years the only psychoanalyst in Indianapolis, became the director of psychotherapy at Norways.[7]

Dr. Dwight Schuster, one of the informants for this chapter, fondly recalled the weekly meetings with patient families and resident staff which were held on Sundays. This instilled a desire in Dr. Schuster to work closely with patient families when he later established his private practice.

A psychiatric nursing program began at Norways in 1947 and this program taught an average of six to eighteen student nurses per year. Betty Ann Countryman was one of the nursing instructors at Norways. Social work student placements began at Norways in 1952. In the early 1950s Norways added a psychiatric library on site. Norways published the *Norways Quarterly*, a newsletter, during the 1950s

Norways Hospital was awarded several grants, including a $50,000 grant from the Indiana Association of Mental Health in 1956. Norways received a Ford Foundation grant of $30,700 in 1957, but this grant money was refunded because the hospital closed. It is unclear what for what purpose these grant monies were intended.[8-9]

Norways had a psychiatry residency that functioned from 1946 until 1957 when the hospital closed. The residency was directed by Philip B. Reed, M.D., who was superintendent during that time period. Dr. Schuster reported that Dr. Reed, as director of Norways residency training, assigned reading to the residents. Some of the better-known residents at Norways included Drs. Nancy Roeske, Richard Kelly Greenbank, W. Arthur Blair, Gordon T. Brown, John P. McNamara, James F. Carlin, Dwight Schuster, Vincent Canganelli, Ray Langdon, Ronald Hull, Julia Thom, and Paul Donner. The total number of residents ranged from one to seven but usually averaged about four. Although Norways was an inpatient psychiatric hospital, residents could see their long-term outpatients in their offices as did Dr. Reed who lived on the hospital grounds.

Medical student externs also worked at Norways. Two well-known Indianapolis area psychiatrists, Drs. Louis Nie and Vincent Alig, were psychiatry externs there. Another very well-known extern at Norways was Arthur B. Richter, M.D. Dr. Richter, born in 1903 in Carroll County, Indiana, attended Indiana University and Harvard University Schools of Medicine. He was the founder and director of the Department of

Electrocardiography at St. Vincent's Hospital. A great benefactor to the Psychiatry Department at Indiana University, he endowed the chair of the Child Psychiatry Department, provided two scholarships in child psychiatry for senior medical students, and endowed the annual Arthur B. Richter Conference in Child Psychiatry.

Wanda Stoops, M.S., a psychologist who performed psychological testing at Norways from 1946 until it closed, fondly recalled a number of the psychiatrists who practiced at Norways. Her favorite was Dr. John Greist. Dr. Philip Reed was a wonderful boss and friend, she said. Dr. Earl Mericle was a light touch for his patients, some of whom persuaded him to discharge them early and then had to be readmitted.

Other well-known staff physicians at Norways included Drs. C. K. Hepburn, Earl Mericle, Dewitt W. Brown, Frank Countryman, Murray DeArmond, John Greist, Sr., Louis W. Nie, George S. Rader, Dwight Schuster, E. Rogers Smith, David L. Phillips, Ronald Hull, George Rader, E. Vernon Hahn, and Robert Bill. According to Dr. Schuster, Earl Mericle always carried the largest patient load and was at the hospital from early in the morning until late at night.

According to Dr. Schuster the range of psychiatric diagnoses at Norways was comparable to that seen in most psychiatric hospitals today, including schizophrenia, manic depressive illness, and psychotic depression. Psychiatry residents worked with all of the patients at Norways but worked extremely closely with Dr. Reed and his private patients. Mrs. Stoops added that she saw a number of cases of postpartum depression, patients with alcoholism, several cases of bromide poisoning, and a few brain injured patients.

Mrs. Stoops mentioned that when the sixty-bed addition was added to Norways, most of the patients housed there were on some form of "shock" therapy, including electroconvulsive therapy, metrazol convulsion therapy, and insulin coma therapy. Orange juice was used to bring patients out of their insulin comas. According to Mrs. Stoops, kitchen workers had to squeeze "mountains" of oranges by hand. When frozen concentrated orange juice was first brought on the market, it was quickly embraced as a great labor-saving product. Early concentrates, however, induced acute gastroenteritis in the patients because of a high concentration of orange peel. Subsequently, concentrated orange juice was abandoned for a brief period until higher quality of orange juice concentrated could be produced.

In 1947 the yearly number of patient days was 10,234 and by 1956 it was 20,449. By the time Norways closed in 1957, the per diem rate was

$28.50, which compared to a $25 a day rate for a psychiatric bed at a general hospital.

During the 1950s Norways found itself in increasing competition for patients with Methodist Hospital. Prior to the opening of the C Psychiatric Wing at Methodist in 1952, psychiatric patients were housed on the 1 B unit on the ground floor. Over time, twelve million dollars was raised for the construction of the new C Wing at Methodist. Although Larue D. Carter Memorial Hospital opened in 1952, this new public psychiatric hospital posed no competition for Norways' private psychiatric patients.

Despite the competition with Methodist, plans were made for the construction of a new Norways Hospital which was to be located just north of Methodist Hospital and was to share facilities and training with Methodist. The new Norways planned to contain one hundred beds, include a residence hall for fifty nurses and was to receive support from the Indianapolis Hospital Development Corporation. Its cost was estimated at 1.6 million dollars.[10-11]

However, because of stiff competition with Methodist for patients, the death knell had sounded for Norways. The patient census was running at only seventy-five percent by the mid-1950s. Norways was closed on October 1, 1957. The land on which Norways was situated was donated to the Marion County Child Guidance Clinic. Proceeds from the sale of Norways were given to the Indiana University School of Medicine Department of Psychiatry. The remaining patients at Norways were moved to Methodist Hospital and the Wabash Valley Sanitarium in Lafayette, Indiana where Dr. Reed relocated.[12-15]

## Methodist Hospital

Methodist Hospital originally opened in April 1908. The first psychiatric patients were housed on the 1 B unit on the ground floor of Methodist Hospital. In the early 1950s Methodist Hospital was the recipient of twelve million dollars from a capital fund campaign through the Indianapolis Hospital Development Corporation Association. Of this sum, $1,400,000 was used to construct a new C-Wing for psychiatric patients. It was opened in June 1959.[1-2] This C-Wing was originally developed to house one hundred seven patients Although a similar unit was planned for private psychiatric patients at Larue D. Carter Memorial Hospital, this plan was never implemented.

The C-Wing contained several units, including a "constant-care unit," a six-bed unit for acutely disturbed patients in the back of the closed unit. The C-Wing contained an occupational therapy department, dining rooms, lounges, and rooms to administer electroconvulsive therapy. Patient rooms contained one, two, or four.

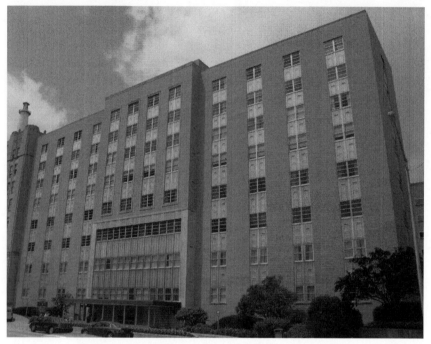

C-Wing, Methodist Hospital, Indianapolis, Indiana

With the opening of new units in the C-Wing, Methodist Hospital became the largest psychiatric service in a non-governmental general hospital in the United States. The final forty-one-bed unit was opened in C-Wing in June 1968. This brought the total number of psychiatric beds at Methodist to one hundred fifty-nine. In all thirty-four private physicians were practicing at Methodist in 1968. The hospital charge for psychiatric care at Methodist in 1968 varied between fifty-one to fifty-five dollars per day.[3]

In April 2010 Methodist Hospital announced plans to tear down the old C-wing and build a new three hundred seventy-five to five hundred million dollar patient care tower which would contain one hundred seventy-five to two hundred fifty patient beds. Construction is to begin in 2012.

## CHAPTER 6

# State Developmental Centers

"In the matter of feeblemindedness of James Carl Sullivan.
Whereas, the proceedings necessary to entitle James Carl
Sullivan to be admitted into the Muscatatuck State School
as a patient, have been had according to law."

Evan West. Jimmy Sullivan: Two boys.
*Indianapolis Monthly*,
Vol. 29, December, 2005, p. 124.

As of 2007 all of the state developmental centers in Indiana had been closed. These centers originated with the bold nineteenth century premise that the developmentally challenged were better off in separate institutions than housed in jails, poor houses, and insane asylums. However, the late twentieth century brought about the ideas of mainstreaming the developmentally challenged in schools and community placement so that there was no longer a need for large state institutions to house them.

The move from state institutions to the community has not been without its problems. Although the move has been a success for many patients,[1] a number of patients simply were moved to developmental disability units at other state hospitals. In addition, deaths of those moved into the community have occurred.[2]

## Fort Wayne Developmental Center

When it opened in 1879 the Fort Wayne Developmental Center was housed in a special wing of the Soldier's and Sailor's Home in Knightstown, Indiana. After a fire in 1886, it moved temporarily to the Eastern Hospital for the Insane in Richmond. It was finally relocated to Fort Wayne and opened in for patients 1890.

The original Fort Wayne site on State Street, originally consisting of fifty-four acres, was purchased on May 19, 1887 for ten thousand dollars from W.L. Carnahan. The main part of the administration building was designed by Fort Wayne architects and cost $37,027.05. Building proceeded over the next several years and added east and west wings to the administration building, laundry, cold storage building bakery, boiler house, electric light plant, school, fever hospital, gymnasium, and an industrial arts building.[1-2] The first superintendent at the Fort Wayne site was John G. Blake.

The 1887 law creating the Indiana School for Feeble-Minded Youth in Fort Wayne defined Feeble-minded as "idiotic, epileptic, and paralytic children."[1] The children were divided into two classes, industrial and custodial. The industrial class of children was taught a trade. The boys were taught "shoe-making, carpentry, mattress making, gardening, farming, brick making, tailoring, woodworking, painting, and upholstering" and the girls were taught "housework, cooking, canning, dining room work, knitting, crocheting, embroidery, dressmaking, loom weaving, laundry, and piano."[1]

During the first through third grades children were taught reading, writing, and arithmetic. The sexes were separated. Children were expected to attend religious instruction on Sundays.

In 1893 several plots of land were purchased in order to start a colony farm. Food produced at the farm was used to feed the school's residents. A brickyard was established on the colony farm. One of the "brickyard reports" indicated that in one year nine boys, working under a hired foreman, produced 250,000 bricks in one year. In 1903 an additional 414 acres of farmland was purchased for the farm colony.

By 1898 children with epilepsy represented twenty-eight percent of the school's enrollment. Epilepsy accounted for at least seventy of the school's deaths. A cemetery was established on the State Street site in which to bury indigent patients.

Enrollment gradually increased over the years. At least three hundred children were transferred to the school when it first opened. By 1906 enrollment had increased to 1,035. By 1937 enrollment was 2,267. Enrollment reached a peak of 2,599 in the late 1960s. Over a twenty year period beginning in the mid-1970s enrollment rapidly decreased to less than five hundred.

The first thirty years of the twentieth century saw much construction. Cottages, a cold storage building, an ice plant, new hospital, dairy barn with silos, and a piggery were constructed. The Black Hawk Farm, consisting of 339 acres, was purchased. The name of the school was changed to the Fort Wayne State School in 1931.

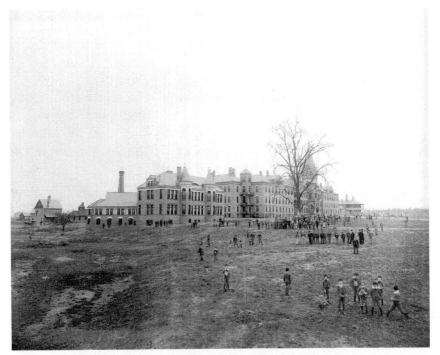

Fort Wayne State School,
photo courtesy of Indiana State Archives, Commission
on Public Records. All rights reserved.

Sterilizations were performed at the school. In 1930 only one female was sterilized. By 1934 this number had risen to fifty-three women and fifty men.[1] This pace finally began dropping by the early 1950s as only nine women and sixteen men were sterilized in the year ending in June 30, 1952.[3]

In 1938 thirty-six academic classes were conducted daily at the Fort Wayne State School. School subjects included arithmetic, reading, spelling, writing, hygiene, history, social studies, and nature. No class size exceeded twelve children.

During World War II the Fort Wayne State School suffered from a shortage of money and employees as did all of the other state institutions for the mentally ill and developmentally disabled. One annual report in the mid 1940s listed only two RNs for 2,363 patients.

In 1956 Bernard Dolnick was appointed superintendent. What followed over the next decade was nothing short of remarkable. One of his first actions was to get rid of the jail cells, whipping straps, leg irons, and strait jackets which had been used for restraint and corporal punishment. This action was no doubt prompted by the banning of corporal punishment by State Mental Health Commissioner Margaret Morgan, M.D., on November 17, 1956.

Superintendent Dolnick made plans to move the entire facility over the next several years to the Oak Park Colony which was further east. This new site was originally approved by the 1955 Indiana General Assembly and was under the leadership of Mental Health Commissioner Margaret Morgan, M.D.[4] Plans for the new site came about largely because of overcrowding of patients in the old facility where one room was crammed so tightly with twenty-seven beds that residents had to scramble over each other to reach their own bed. The plan was a also response to many teachers at the school leaving for higher paying positions elsewhere.[5]

In 1960 many of the school's residents moved from the East State Street site to this new Parker Place site at the intersection of Stelhorn and St. Joe Road.[6] Here residents were housed in cottages instead of large hospital wards. New buildings were constructed including a hospital, dormitories, power plant and school. In the mid 1960s a two million dollar vocational training and maintenance building was added to the new campus.

In 1966 Ora R. Ackerman, Ed.D., became the next superintendent. He carried forth on plans to expend the facility at the new site and begin the demolition of old buildings at the State Street site. Five new residential buildings were constructed at the new site. A "club program" with Boy Scout, Girl Scout, and 4-H groups was begun. A Foster Grandparent Program was initiated as was a new job training program. In 1977 the Fort Wayne State School and Training Center was certified as an Intermediate Care Facility for the Mentally Retarded. A new activity center was constructed. This building housed a swimming pool, gymnasium, library, audio-visual studio, auditorium, canteen, vocational training areas, clinics, beauty and barber shop, and clothing store.

In 1985 the facility again changed its name to the Fort Wayne State Developmental Center. In 1986 it was accredited by the Accreditation Council for Services to Developmentally Disabled Persons. In 1988 Dr. Ackerman stepped down from his position as superintendent.

Over the next twenty years there were five acting superintendents with the exception of Ajit Kumar Mukherjee, Ph.D., who served as superintendent from 1991-2001. In 2005 Liberty Healthcare of Bala Cynwyd, Pennsylvania was brought in to manage the Fort Wayne Developmental Center until it closed in June 2007.

## New Castle State Developmental Center

Ohio was the first state to establish a separate state institution devoted to the treatment of individuals with epilepsy. Known as the Ohio Hospital for Epileptics, it was established in 1890 in Gallopolis, Ohio. Indiana's hospital for epileptics, originally the Indiana Village for Epileptics, was founded in 1906. Dr. George Edenharter, while he was superintendent at Central State Hospital, was largely responsible for the establishment of the Indiana Village for Epileptics. It was established because epilepsy was originally believed to be a mental illness, but persons with epilepsy had been inappropriately housed in state hospitals for the insane. Renamed the New Castle State Hospital, it eventually began to treat developmentally challenged adults and was renamed the New Castle State Developmental Center.[1]

Competition was fierce for a location to establish this new state hospital. Many Indiana communities, including Greencastle, New Castle, Orange County, Winamac, Franklin, Elkhart, and Plymouth made bids for the hospital, but the Indiana State Legislature finally settled on the "New Castle Compromise," whereby land was bought at a moderate price and the hospital was more centrally located.

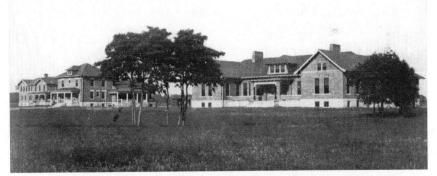

New Castle Colony 2: White, Employee, and Baker Buildings
photo courtesy of Indiana State Archives, Commission
on Public Records. All rights reserved.

Walter C. VanNuys, M.D., was the first superintendent of the Indiana Village for Epileptics. In 1946 there were 1,036 patient beds housed in cottage style buildings.[2] In 1945 the facility was situated on thirteen hundred acres, seven hundred of which were used for farming. Like other state hospitals in Indiana at the time, New Castle raised food from its farm program. This program raised seventy percent of food consumed there including potatoes, beans, tomatoes, corn, apples, beets, peas, carrots, strawberries, milk, beef, pork, butter, cheese, and poultry. Many of these foods were canned or preserved.[3] William Murray, M.D., was another of New Castle's superintendents. Serving from 1959 until 1971, he left to become one of Indiana's Commissioners of Mental Health.

The original site of the Indiana Village for Epileptics contained eleven abandoned farm houses. Dr. VanNuys originally lived in one of these farm houses. In 1907 the first residents were fifty-five men who were housed in two cottages.

Women were not admitted until 1925. Prior to 1925 women with epilepsy who became violent were housed in either jails or state mental institutions. Women were accepted in groups of twenty in 1925 and began occupying eight new cottage style buildings which had been constructed along with a new administration building, receiving center, laundry, power house, dining hall, hospital, and industrial building.[4] When construction was complete, men were housed on the east side of Blue River Valley and women on the west side. Patients were segregated according to age and developmental abilities.

Prior to 1953 when eight-hour shifts were established for employees, most of the cottages had a married couple and a housekeeper who were on call twenty-four hours a day, six days a week. A few cottages were supervised by single women. Other employees worked twelve-hour shifts.[1]

The security force at New Castle had an interesting job. In 1961 security officers disposed of thirty-one stray dogs and fifty-one stray cats in addition to their regular duties of returning twenty-three AWOL patients and issuing thirty parking tickets.[1]

The New Castle State Developmental Center closed in 1998 and all but three buildings were demolished, making way for the construction of the New Castle Correctional Facility.[5]

## Muscatatuck State Developmental Center

The Muscatatuck State Developmental Center, originally named the Indiana Farm Colony for Feeble Minded Youth, opened in 1920. It was located on 1,814 acres of land near Butlerville in Jennings County. By 1940 this institution had grown to twenty-one hundred acres with eleven hundred of them under cultivation. Originally only mentally retarded males over age sixteen were admitted. In 1933 the colony started admitting women and in 1937 its name was changed to the Muscatatuck Colony. In 1941 its name was changed again to the Muscatatuck State School. At that time it began accepting both male and female patients over age six from the southern half of Indiana and in 1949 it began accepting children under the age of six.[1]

The first male patients at Muscatatuck came from the Indiana School for Feeble Minded Youth in Fort Wayne and the Indiana Reformatory. These boys and men lived in three farm houses on the property. In the early 1920s three dormitories were built, the Aitkenhead Colony Building in 1921, the Keller Building in 1922, and the Scott Building in 1924. Each of these buildings housed sixty patients who worked on the farm, blacksmith shop, canning factory, or the stone quarry. When girls and women were admitted, two new dormitories were added, Tyler and Madison Halls. Other new buildings included a laundry building, plumbing/electrical building, and carpentry/paint building. As younger children began to be admitted, the focus changed from vocational to educational programs.[2]

In 1938 construction of eighteen new buildings began, funded by a grant from the Public Works Administration. These buildings included a school, seven new dormitories, two infirmaries, four staff residences, a service building, and a farm colony building. All of these buildings were constructed in the Art Deco style.

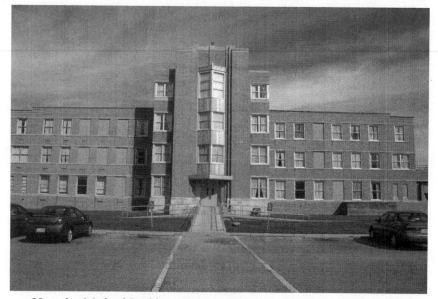

Hingeley Medical Building, Muscatatuck State Developmental Center
photo courtesy of Indiana State Archives, Commission
on Public Records. All rights reserved.

In 1940 a new hospital building was constructed in response to the recognition that a number of physical conditions, such as cretinism (a congenital form of hypothyroidism), mongolianism (Down's syndrome), hydrocephaly (water on the brain), microcephaly (small head), and spasticity (cerebral palsy), were recognized as causing developmental delays. Persons with intellectual disabilities in the 1940s were classified as idiot, imbecile, and moron in order of increasing intelligence.[3]

During the tenure of Donald Jolly, M.D., as superintendent from 1957-67, a chapel was built on the grounds. Five sixteen-bed cottages were built for higher functioning patients in addition to two other cottages for less capable patients. One of the more interesting construction projects was jokingly referred to as "Jolly's folly" while it was under construction. It consisted of a twenty by forty foot wooden floored and sided contraption that could be raised and lowered in the small lake on the grounds so that patients could safely swim. It was also referred to as the "corn crib."

Over time, the census at Muscatatuck grew from six hundred residents in 1937 to a population of thirteen hundred in 1941. In 1963 the population was 2,048 with a very large waiting list for admission. Clearly this institution filled a need in Indiana.

Like other state mental health and developmental disabilities facilities, Muscatatuck was not immune from scandal, some deserved and some undeserved. In 1957 Indiana governor Harold Handley ordered an investigation by Indiana's Counter-Subversive Study Commission into possible communist infiltration at the facility. At the same time a separate grand jury investigation revealed sexual "immorality" and an increase of pregnancies among the Muscatatuck residents, which was believed caused by inadequate staff supervision.[4]

Ms Angie Eckstein, longtime social worker at Larue Carter Memorial Hospital, recalled many fond memories of having worked at Muscatatuck. In 1954 Angie began working there part-time while still a social work student at Indiana University in Indianapolis. She continued working there until 1957 when she moved to Iowa for a few years to work at the Glenwood State School. When she arrived at Muscatatuck, Alfred Sasser, Jr., M.D., was superintendent. During his reign at Muscatatuck Dr. Sasser had modernized the facility with many improvements including hiring many new professional staff and installing a state-of-the-art speech and audiology laboratory. All patients received intellectual testing.

When Angie arrived, about two thousand patients were at Muscatatuck, including a nursery full of infants. Patients had a wide range of intellectual capabilities. Angie recalled that she attended the burial of one of her patients in the cemetery of the state school; he had disappeared one day and was found months later on the school's grounds. While employed at Muscatatuck, Angie lived first in an employee dormitory and later in an apartment with two other employees. Rent was cheap, about twenty-five dollars a month, and food was excellent and plentiful, thanks to an employee point system which allowed workers to purchase food at the school's grocery store. She remembered the school as being entirely self-sufficient with laundry, workshops, water supply, powerhouse, etc.

As the times changed, fewer and fewer individuals were sent to live in Indiana's developmental centers because of increased funding for treatment in the community in group homes and nursing homes. The story of the discharge of Jimmy Sullivan from the Muscatatuck State Developmental Center is particularly poignant, because not all discharges from our state institutions have been successful, despite what politicians and state administrators would have us to believe.[5]

Jimmy Sullivan was born was born in 1946. He was normal in every way except for delayed speech. At age two and a half, he sustained a head injury when hit by a pickup truck. By age five and a half his vocabulary was only fifty words. His behavior in kindergarten was uncontrollable. On the advice of physicians at age six, Jimmy was sent to Muscatatuck by the court. Jimmy lived the next fifty years at Muscatatuck. He had fits of anger, tore off his clothes at times, and was diagnosed with bipolar disorder, a psychotic condition. He had a job shredding recyclable paper, but spent most of his time drawing in the arts and crafts center. In 2001 Indiana governor Frank O'Bannon announced the closure of Muscatatuck to take place in 2005. Jimmy was sent to a group home in North Vernon, Indiana. Jimmy lived not quite three months in that home. He tragically died at a McDonald's restaurant when he choked after he gulped hamburger and french-fries despite having been fed pureed food at Muscatatuck for many years previously because of the condition of his teeth. Between 2001 and 2005 at least four of Muscatatuck's longtime residents have died in accidents while in private care.

The Muscatatuck State Developmental Center was closed in June 2005 and in 2009 its grounds became the Muscatatuck Urban Training Center, the United States Army's urban warfare training site.[6]

## Northern Indiana State Developmental Center

Built on eleven acres of land near Notre Dame University in 1950, the Northern Indiana State Developmental Center began life as the Northern Indiana Children's Hospital in South Bend. The hospital was built at a cost of one million eight hundred thousand dollars and had one hundred beds. Originally it housed children with multiple physical handicaps, such as polio. Because of competition with Riley Hospital in Indianapolis, its early daily population was only eighteen to twenty patients. Eventually it became a developmental center for the mentally retarded. It was closed in 1998.[1-2]

## Silvercrest Children's Developmental Center

Silvercrest is worthy of mention if only because it is an architectural gem built in the art deco style. Originally opened in New Albany, Indiana in 1941 as a regional tuberculosis hospital, Silvercrest was converted into a children's developmental center in 1974. The one hundred fifty bed hospital was a one million dollar WPA project built on a high ridge in the beautiful Silver Hills region overlooking New Albany and the Ohio River. Built of Indiana limestone and tan brick, it had translucent glass block windows at either end. The six-story main hospital building was built on a forty-two acre site. All patient rooms were individual and the hospital was complete with clinical laboratories and surgical suites.[1]

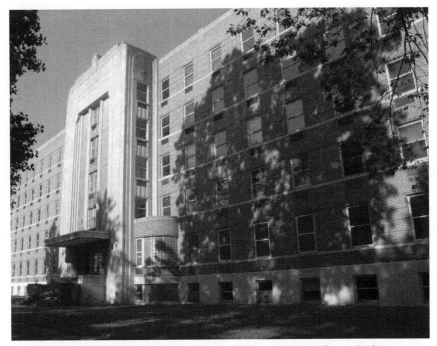

Silvercrest Children's Developmental Center, New Albany, Indiana

Purchased in 1924 for six thousand five hundred dollars, the land for the site came from the Hardy farm on Old Vincennes Road. Fundraising efforts over the next twelve years made possible a twenty-bed tuberculosis sanitarium to be built on the site. In 1938 the Indiana General Assembly passed a bill establishing a Southern Indiana Tuberculosis Hospital. New Albany was one of thirteen communities which competed for the location of this hospital, which originally served a forty-county area.[2]

In 1974 Silvercrest was converted to a children's developmental center. Over the next twenty-five years, Silvercrest served two thousand multiply handicapped children, thirty percent of them having over three or more major disabilities.[3] It was closed down in 2006 by the administration of Governor Mitchell Daniels. Although employees and patients' families waged a fierce court battle to save the hospital, its fate was sealed by efforts to relocate the treatment of the developmentally disabled in the communities in which they live. In 2007 a New Albany developer purchased the land and buildings with plans to turn the property into housing for senior citizens.[4]

CHAPTER 7

# Correctional Facilities

"Two wrongs don't make a right,
but they make a good excuse."

Thomas Szasz,
*The Second Sin*, 1973

As we have seen from the beginning of the Indiana Territory in 1800, county jails have never been good places in which to house or treat the mentally ill. In addition, state prisons have not been good places to house and treat incarcerated criminals who are mentally ill. After all, correctional officers are not trained mental health professionals. In Indiana it wasn't until 1910 that the Indiana State Prison had a special unit for the treatment of mentally ill prisoners. Finally in 1955 Indiana opened a separate facility within a mental hospital in which to treat these prisoners.

## Indiana State Prison

Prior to the opening in 1952 of the Northern Indiana Insane Hospital, later known as Norman Beatty Memorial Hospital, the criminally insane were housed in a three-story structure built in 1910 known as the Insane Criminal Division at the Indiana State Prison in Michigan City, Indiana. Even some mentally ill patients deemed too difficult to control in other state hospitals were sometimes housed there. For example, runaways from state hospitals were sometimes adjudged criminal violators and sent to this Indiana State Prison unit. In 1953 there existed two wards of violent criminally mentally ill men at the Indiana Sate Prison. These two massive wards held a total of two hundred thirty patients. In spite of the large number of mentally ill criminals, there had never been a full-time psychiatrist at the Indiana State Prison. Nonviolent patients housed at the

Indiana State Prison slept in crowded rooms containing bunk beds. There was little or no treatment provided.

In January 1954 a process began to transfer the criminally mentally ill to the new Norman Beatty Hospital in nearby Westville, Indiana. At this new hospital they were placed in a four million five hundred thousand dollar Maximum Security Division.[1]

## Norman Beatty Memorial Hospital

Prior to the opening of the Norman Beatty Memorial Hospital, initially known as the Northern Indiana Insane Hospital, persons found not guilty by reason of insanity were held at the Indiana State Prison in Michigan City. This situation was inappropriate because a state prison or county jails were inappropriate places to house such individuals, not to mention that the staff at Indiana's ninety-two county jails and the Indiana State Prison was not trained in treating mentally ill individuals. In addition, because of overcrowding in Indiana's other state mental hospitals, severely out-of-control mentally ill individuals were often housed in county jails until they could be civilly committed. These patients had to wait an average of at least two weeks before they could be hospitalized and sometimes they languished in county jails for months before a hospital bed became available. Therefore, Governor Ralph Gates announced in 1946 that land in LaPorte County near Westville had been purchased for $136,660 for a new mental hospital. Approximately one hundred fifty thousand dollars had been appropriated by the 1945 Indiana State Legislature to buy land for this new hospital.[1-2]

However, it was not until July 1949 that the cornerstone was laid for this new hospital by the next Indiana governor, Henry Schricker. The main hospital and administration building were to cost two million dollars. Thirty buildings were planned on the 1,322 acre site and the total cost for the entire complex would eventually be twenty-two million dollars. The complex was expected to house four thousand individuals. Other hospital structures were to include a water system, sewage treatment plant, electrical plant, laundry, service buildings, warehouses, chapel, auditorium, dining rooms, dormitories, and living quarters for employees. Construction was to last until 1955 and ultimately this new hospital would increase the capacity of Indiana's public mental hospital system by thirty percent for a total of nine thousand individuals. Final plans called for the facility to house six hundred fifty criminals in a separate enclosed area. The remainder of the facility was reserved for civilly committed patients.[3]

In 1952 the name of Northern Indiana Insane Hospital was changed to Norman M. Beatty Hospital in order to honor a former director of the Indiana State Board of Health. Dr. Beatty was a pioneer in hospital sanitation and was a strong activist for improving Indiana's mental health facilities. The hospital's first superintendent was Herbert McMahan, M.D., and the assistant superintendent was Wallace Van Den Bosch, M.D. Dr. McMahan initially predicted a sixty-five percent cure rate.

On the first day of admission to the hospital patients were interviewed, given a physical exam, and assigned to a treatment team. On the second day the treatment team presented the case history and decided on a treatment plan. There were plans to use sedative medications, electroconvulsive therapy, insulin coma therapy, carbon dioxide therapy, and narcosynthesis. Restraints were forbidden.[4-6]

In contrast to civilly committed patients, the criminally insane were housed in the Maximum Security Division, a separate unit on the grounds of the hospital. This unit was divided into eight two-story buildings. One was a medical hospital, the second housed the elderly, a third housed maximum security cases, and a fourth housed a hydrotherapy unit. Another building housed recreational facilities and the remaining three buildings were dormitories.[7]

Almost from its inception Beatty Hospital had problems. First and foremost was the low pay for state hospital attendants. In 1952 Beatty attendants averaged one hundred thirty dollars per month. Registered nurses were paid two hundred dollars a month.[8]

The second superintendent of Norman Beatty Hospital, Wallace Van Den Bosch, M.D., quit his position in September 1956 after serving five years. He and then Indiana governor George Craig had a fundamental disagreement over who should control the hospital's Maximum Security Division. Dr. Van Den Bosch felt that Beatty Hospital should be controlled entirely by the superintendent, not a warden as Governor Craig proposed. This confrontation between Governor Craig and Superintendent Van Den Bosch had grown out of a series of escapes from the Maximum Security Division.[9]

A little over eleven years later in December 1967, David P. Morton, M.D., third superintendent of Norman Beatty Hospital, resigned. He had had problems in recruiting qualified hospital staff and hoped that his resignation and retirement would draw attention to the problem.[10]

From 1977-79 the patients at Norman Beatty Hospital were gradually transferred to other state hospitals. The facility was renamed the Westville Correctional Facility and became part of the Indiana Department of Corrections in 1979.

With the closing of Norman Beatty Hospital, the care of mentally ill prisoners reverted to the numerous separate correctional facilities within Indiana. It wasn't until 2002 that a separate facility was built for mentally ill offenders. This facility, the New Castle Correctional Facility, costing $118,000,000, was built on the grounds of the old New Castle State Hospital. In addition to housing the mentally ill on special units, other medium security offenders are housed here. From the onset, this facility has had problems in obtaining and keeping staff capable of treating the mentally ill. For example, in 2004 because of budget shortfalls, New Castle, built to house 1,296 inmates, only held 375 inmates.[11]

## Chapter 8

# Community Mental Health Centers

"We as a Nation have long neglected the mentally ill and the mentally retarded. This neglect must end, if our nation is to live up to its own standards of compassion and dignity and achieve the maximum use of its manpower....

We must act to bestow the full benefits of our society on those who suffer from mental disabilities; to prevent the occurrence of mental illness and mental retardation wherever and whenever possible; to provide for early diagnosis and continuous and comprehensive care, in the community, of those suffering from these disorders; to stimulate improvements in the level of care given the mentally disabled in our State and private institutions, and to reorient those programs to a community-centered approach; to reduce, over a number of years, and by hundreds of thousands, the persons confined to these institutions; to retain in and return to the community the mentally ill and mentally retarded, and then to restore and revitalize their lives through better health programs and strengthened educational and rehabilitation services...

To achieve these important ends, I urge that the Congress favorably act upon the foregoing recommendations."

President John F. Kennedy's speech to
Congress on February 5, 1963.

In 1963 the United States Congress passed the Community Mental Health Centers Act and it was signed into law by President John F. Kennedy. This act enabled individual states to obtain federal grants to support the construction of community mental health centers. Each center was to serve a catchment area population of between 75,000 and 250,000 individuals. In addition each center was to provide five essential services which included inpatient hospitalization, partial hospitalization, outpatient care, emergency services, and consultation services. Accordingly the Indiana Department of Mental Health, in collaboration with local communities and chapters of the Mental Health Association, began the planning to establish not-for-profit corporations which became community mental health centers.[1]

In 1965 Indiana passed a law authorizing Indiana counties "to furnish financial assistance for constructing and operating community mental health centers."[2] However, it wasn't until 1969 that the Midtown Community Mental Health Center became the first community mental health center to open in Indiana. Midtown, as it became to be known, was situated at Marion County General Hospital in Indianapolis, Indiana. Over the next fifteen years another twenty-nine community mental health centers were opened in Indiana.

During the administration of President Jimmy Carter the Mental Health Systems Act was passed. This act required additional psychiatric services, including screening, child and adolescent, rape crisis, alcohol and drug abuse, and residential and elderly services.

One of the most drastic changes in the operation of Indiana's community mental health centers came about in the mid 1990s. A "gatekeeper" function was established so that only community mental health centers would be allowed to refer mentally ill patients to Indiana's remaining state mental hospitals. An exception for this rule was allowed for Carter Hospital's Research Service. Nearly all patients are now civilly committed, with the exception those who are incompetent to stand trial or have been adjudged not guilty by reason of insanity. These individuals are referred by the courts to the Division of Mental Health where decisions are made on placement on a case by case basis.

Since most of Indiana's community mental health centers were established after 1975, this chapter will describe only four of the earliest community mental health centers established in Indiana. Due to the recent economic downturn some community mental health centers have merged with others and some have even had to lay off treatment personnel.

## Midtown Community Mental Health Center

Midtown Community Mental Health Center opened in November 1969 in the B and C Wings of Marion County General Hospital. Of the ninety-four beds in the new psychiatric wing, half were allocated to Midtown. Space was provided for outpatient treatment and occupational and recreational therapies. The original catchment area for Midtown included most of Marion County's Center Township and areas west including Speedway.[3] Over the next several decades Midtown expanded away from Wishard Hospital into a number of satellite clinics and residential facilities. A twenty-four-hour crisis team was formed to staff the crisis intervention unit and the hospital's emergency room. Addictions services were provided as were services for children and adolescents. Adult daycare was provided at several Midtown sites. Home visits and treatment for the homeless were begun. Midtown was staffed with its own employees and the center was used and continues to be used for the training of psychiatry residents, psychology interns, social workers, and medical students from Indiana University School of Medicine.

## Katherine Hamilton Mental Health Center

Vigo County resident Katherine Hamilton was unhappy with her sister's mental health treatment and through her volunteer efforts fought for years to improve treatment of the mentally ill. Her efforts resulted in the opening of the Vigo County Adult and Child Guidance Clinic and numerous other mental health initiatives in Vigo County. Because of her tremendous efforts, it was natural that the community mental health center that opened in Terre Haute, Indiana in 1971 would be named after her. Since its opening the Hamilton Center has grown to six hundred employees and has satellite clinics in nine other counties.

## Oaklawn Community Mental Health Center

Oaklawn grew out of a vision of the Mennonite Central Committee in Ohio, Indiana, Michigan, and Illinois for the need for more Christian mental health care in the region. This vision resulted in the opening of Oaklawn in Elkhart in 1963. Otto Klassen, M.D., was its first medical director. With the passage of the Community Mental Health Centers Act, Oaklawn officials made plans to become a community mental health center which opened in 1973. Currently Oaklawn has about five hundred fifty employees and provides mental health services in Indiana and Michigan.

## Gallahue Community Mental Health Center

Gallahue Community Mental Health Center was the second community mental health center to be established in Marion County. Gallahue was named after Edward F. Gallahue who was born near Indianapolis, Indiana in 1902. Born in a family punctuated by mental illness, alcoholism, and divorce, he and his brother founded the American States Insurance Company. He was extremely active in civic and religious affairs and was a valuable contributor to the Indiana Mental Health Association. He went on to sponsor conferences on mental health and religion at the Menninger's Clinic in Topeka, Kansas and the Princeton Seminary in New Jersey.

Besides the east side of Marion County, Gallahue's catchment area included Hancock, Madison, and Shelby Counties to the east of Marion County. Gallahue's services were launched in July 1974. By 1976 its staff had grown to sixty.[4] Currently Gallahue offers the full range of mental health services required by federal law and also serves as a training site for psychiatry residents and psychology interns from Indiana University School of Medicine.

## Other Community Mental Health Centers in Indiana

In 2010 the other community mental health centers in Indiana include the following listed alphabetically by the town where the Community Mental Health Center's home office is located:

Avon – Cummins Mental Health Center
Bloomington – Cornerstone of Indiana University
Carmel – BehaviorCorp
Evansville – Southwestern Behavioral Healthcare
Fort Wayne – Park Center
Gary – Edgewater Systems
Indianapolis – Adult and Child Mental Health Center
Jasper – Southern Hills Counseling Center
Jeffersonville – Lifespring
Kendallville – Northeastern Center
Kokomo – Howard Community Hospital Psychiatric Services
Lawrenceburg – Community Mental Health Center
Logansport – Four County Counseling Center
Marion – Grant-Blackford Mental Health
Merrillville – Southlake Community Mental Health Center

Michigan City – Swanson Center
Muncie – Meridian Services
Richmond – Dunn Mental Health Center
South Bend – Madison Center
Valparaiso – Porter-Starke Services
Vincennes – Samaritan Center
West Lafayette – Wabash Valley Hospital

CHAPTER 9

# Psychiatric Organizations

Prosecutor: Dr. Smith, you are making some claim that
you are an expert on this matter of insanity?
Dr. Smith: Yes sir, I do.
Prosecutor: What are your qualifications?
Dr. Smith: Well, in the first place, I was born in a hospital
for the insane!

Paul H. Buchanan, Jr.
Courting disaster:
Recollections of an Indiana judge
about Dr. E. Rogers Smith.
*Indiana Medicine*, 78(8), 1985, p. 660.

We have chosen to discuss only three representative psychiatric organizations: the Indiana Division of Mental Health and Addictions, the Indiana Psychiatric Society, and Mental Health of America, formerly the Indiana Mental Health Association. There are a great many other psychiatric and psychological associations including numerous other professional groups, hospital organizations, family and self-help groups, etc., but we chose the three of most relevance to psychiatrists.

## Division of Mental Health and Addictions

The governmental agency responsible for mental health in Indiana has undergone a number of name changes during its history in the twentieth century. In 1945 the Indiana Council on Mental Health was established to oversee state mental hospitals.[1] Originally the Council had five members: a judge from a circuit court, a physician in general practice, a psychiatric physician with medical school teaching experience, the chief executive officer of the State Welfare Department, and the chief executive officer of the State Board of Health. In 1953 the Council was made part of the Indiana State Department of Health, but in 1961 it was separated from this agency and was renamed the Department of Mental Health.[2]

The original members of the Indiana Council for Mental Health included Larue D. Carter, M.D., Norman M. Beatty, M.D., Clifford L. Williams, M.D., Judge John Morris of the Henry County Circuit Court, Otto F. Walls, and Leroy Burney, M.D. Unfortunately Dr. Carter died on January 22, 1946 just twenty-one days after taking office. He was replaced by Clifford L. Williams, M.D., a psychiatrist. Initially the Council visited all of the state mental and disability facilities. They found that the treatment offered differed markedly from facility to facility, but that custodial care predominated. They found that Indiana was far behind in caring for the mentally disturbed. Indiana was thirty-second nationally in the number of persons per 100,000 population institutionalized (262.2), thirty-ninth in expenditures at $212.91 per patient per year, and thirtieth in number of employees per one thousand patients (126.8). Indiana had one physician for every 374 patients when the national average was one per 319 and the American Psychiatric Association recommended one physician per one hundred fifty patients at the time. There was one social worker for every 2,248 patients whereas the national average was one per 1,015. Tuberculosis was a problem and some facilities did not offer isolation for infected patients.[3]

Originally the Department of Mental Health was housed at Larue Carter Memorial Hospital and included separate divisions for child mental health and mental retardation. After an addictions division was added and the Department of Mental Health became known as the Division of Mental Health and Addictions. Finally in 1991, in order to consolidate and better integrate the delivery of human services, the Indiana General Assembly established the Family and Social Services Administration, a super-agency to oversee five care divisions. These divisions include: 1) Division of Family Resources, 2) Office of Medicaid Policy and Planning, 3) Division of Disability and Rehabilitative Services, 4) Division of Mental Health and Addiction, and 5) Division of Aging. Currently the Division of Mental Health and Addictions oversees the six state psychiatric hospitals and the mental health provider network composed primarily of community mental health centers.

From 1953 to 1981 the commissioners of the Department/Division of Mental Health included[1]:

| Margaret E. Morgan, M.D. | 1953-1957 |
| John Southworth, M.D. | 1957-1958 |
| Stuart T. Ginsburg, M.D. | 1958-1966 |
| J.R. Gambill, M.D. | 1966-1967 |
| William F. Sheeley, M.D. | 1967-1969 |
| John U. Keating, M.D. | 1969-1970 |
| William E. Murray | 1970-1981 |

## Indiana Psychiatric Society

### The Earliest Days of Organized Psychiatry in Indiana[1]

The Indiana Psychiatric Society began as a group of psychiatrists, neurologists and neuropsychiatrists known as the Indiana Neuropsychiatric Association (INPA). The earliest beginnings, like those of many organizations are shrouded by the mists of time. Early meetings were either not recorded or records were discarded over time, leaving no written records of the first decade of INPA activity.

Fortunately, several charter members were still alive in 1986. Armed with a tape recorder, a few dictated reminiscences and great determination, I bumped over country roads and snaked through city streets to find them and hear their stories. Drs. John Greist and Philip Reed, psychiatrists involved in early INPA meetings, kindly granted interviews and provided a wealth of information.

First Meeting at French Lick

The November 1937 *ISMA Journal* reported that the eighty-eighth Annual Convention, held from October 4-6, 1937 at French Lick, enjoyed splendid weather and boasted a record attendance of 684 physicians. At this time the ISMA had only a few specialty sections, and none existed for psychiatry or neurology. The American Board of Psychiatry and Neurology had only been founded three years previously and many of its members had been grandfathered/grandmothered in. In 1937, as far as the AMA was concerned, one became a psychiatrist, neurologist, or neuropsychiatrist simply by placing a P, N, or NP after one's name in the AMA Annual Directory.

It was amid this setting that the INPA was born. In a 1978 letter to Philip Morton, M.D., Philip Reed described the meeting that led to the organizational meeting of the INPA:

"Larue Carter had reviewed with several of us in the mid-1930s his pleasure at the steadily growing number of physicians in Indiana whose major field of interest was psychiatry or neurology or, more usually, both. He had suggested to E. Rogers Smith, M.D., that the several who had responded to his mention of a state society might best meet in conjunction with the Indiana State Medical Association annual meeting in French Lick in October 1937. With "Rog" and several others supporting the idea, contacts were made and some six or eight men gathered informally for the discussion. This group, which met on the wide porch at the left of the top of the long flight of steps at the front entrance of the French Lick Springs Hotel, was composed of Drs. Larue Carter, John Hare, Murray DeArmond, Louis P. Harshman, Keith Hepburn, E. Rogers Smith, Clifford Williams, Philip Reed, and possibly one or two others. A half-circle were seated in the high cane-back rockers, the others were seated on or standing near the porch railing. It was quickly decided that the time had come for a state-wide organization of neuropsychiatrists. Larue Carter was asked to issue the call for the organization meeting to be held at Norways Sanitarium as soon as was convenient."

## Organizational Meeting at Norways

The date of this meeting is uncertain but Dr. Reed believed it may have been held in late 1938. "Invitations by phone or letter went out to all the men and women in Indiana who elected to have a P, N, or NP after their names in the AMA Annual Directory, indicating their major field of interest." The majority of the founding members practiced both neurology and psychiatry.

About fifteen physicians gathered on the sun porch at Norways, located at 1820 E. 10th Street in Indianapolis. In this large room, furnished with white painted rattan furniture, Larue Carter called the animate group to order and it was rapidly decided that a statewide society should indeed be formed and that its name was to be the Indiana Neuropsychiatric Association. Larue Carter was the natural choice for President. Phil Reed was elected Secretary-Treasurer. Dr. Carter was directed to appoint a committee of his own choosing to meet with him to draft a constitution and bylaws. The next meeting was to be at the call of the President for discussion of the first draft of the constitution and for a short scientific session.

The substance of this meeting dealt largely with a sharing of opinions about what a neuropsychiatric association in Indiana might do and where meetings might be held. Members mentioned that Indiana is a long state and people like Dr. John Hare (Superintendent of Evansville State Hospital), who was not present at the meeting, and Dr. Louis Harshman (from Ft. Wayne) would need to be accommodated in choosing meeting sites.

## A Colorful and Commanding Group

Those in attendance at the organizational meeting included some commanding and colorful figures. Max Bahr, M.D., Superintendent of Central State Hospital, had lectured at Indiana University School of Medicine in psychiatry and neurology in the 1920s when the psychiatry lectures consisted of two hours on Saturday afternoons in the senior year. He is credited with the following ditty about paresis:

> "Age of twenty, girls aplenty, wit and wine galore,
> Age of thirty, still quite flirty, drinking more and more,
> Age of forty, would be naughty, if he had the vim,
> Age of fifty, got paresis, and that's the end of him!"

Larue D. Carter was a birthright Quaker from Westfield who trained in Indiana, interned at Indianapolis City Hospital and took a two-year internship at Philadelphia General where he became interested in psychiatry and neurology. He served as a house officer under Superintendent Samuel E. Smith, M.D., (fondly known as "Psycho Sam") at Richmond State Hospital. After serving as Division Surgeon for the 38th Division of the Indiana National Guard in 1916, and rising to the command of a base hospital during WW I, he returned to Indianapolis around 1919 and joined Dr. Albert Stern who had founded the Norways Sanitarium. After Dr. Stern died in 1931, Dr. Carter became the Director of Norways Sanitarium. There he lectured to medical students and later conducted a residency training program until his death in 1946. As Dr. Greist put it, among psychiatrists "he just stood out like Mount Olympus." Dr. Reed describes him as a "father figure to most of the psychiatrists in the state in 1937."

Irving Page, M.D., Director of the Lilly Research Ward at Indianapolis City Hospital, was neither psychiatrist nor neurologist and was present by special invitation. He had just returned form several years as Director of the Kaiser Wilhelm Institute in Berlin and had an interest in neurology and psychiatry. In 1938 he had recently published *The Chemistry of the Brain*. At the Norways meeting Frank Hutchins, M.D., commented that he had just read this most fascinating book which set forth many new theories about the nervous system. Turning to Page, he asked, "Do you know anything about it?" "Yes," Page replied, "I wrote it!" Dr. Page later left Indianapolis to join the Cleveland Clinic where he accrued fame for his work in hypertension.

E. Rogers Smith, M.D., primarily a neurologist, who trained at Michigan and taught at Indiana University School of Medicine, was the son of Samuel E. Smith, M.D., Superintendent of Richmond State Hospital. "Rog" was fond of serving as an expert witness and mentioning in court that he was born in an insane asylum. Smith's attachment to Dr. Carter dated from his college days when Dr. Carter's closet at Richmond provided a place to hide alcohol while at home visiting his teetotalling father. "Rog" had a private practice in Indianapolis.

Frank Hutchins, M.D., was a neuropsychiatrist who taught at Indiana University in the 1920s. At the time of this organizational meeting he was approaching retirement and the status of elder-statesman of the group. Philip B. Reed, M.D., had graduated from Indiana University School of Medicine in 1930, interned at Indianapolis City Hospital, and became Assistant Superintendent there in 1932. He received psychiatric training at Norways and was Assistant Director there when INPA was founded. He and his wife's close relationship with the childless Larue and Ann Carter led to the Carter's legal adoption of them.

Also present at this meeting were Drs. Charles Cottingham, Murray DeArmond, Louis Harshman (Ft. Wayne), C. Keith Hepburn, "Jake" Norton (Columbus), Thomas P. Rogers, W. Leland Sharp, and Clifford L. Williams (Superintendent of Logansport State Hospital).

## War and New Hospitals: INPA in the 1940s [2]

The history of INPA during the 1940's was dominated by two events: World War II and the lobby to build new state psychiatric hospitals. The war reduced psychiatric coverage in Indiana to a minimum as numerous physicians joined the military. The psychiatric faculty at Indiana University which numbered six or seven before the war was reduced to two members, Drs. Philip Reed and David Boyd. Regular INPA meetings were prevented, not by a shortage of gasoline or tires, but by time pressures created by the need to cover the psychiatric business of the state with greatly reduced numbers of physicians.

Little information exists about INPA's early meetings. Dr. Reed recalled only two meetings at Norways. Most of the early meetings were held at the Athenaeum in Indianapolis. The first scientific sessions included Dr.

Breutsch's ongoing work at Central State Hospital on the malarial treatment of paresis, reports by the Norway staff on what was then the only insulin coma treatment in the state, and a little later, the first electroconvulsive treatment in Indiana. Dr. Reed also recalled discussion of what might be the most effective sedation of manic patients in light of the new prolonged sleep treatment of mania in use at that time.

INPAs founder and first president, Larue D. Carter, M.D., was a prime mover behind the building of Larue Carter and Norman Beatty Hospitals. His portrait hung in the lobby of the original 1315 West 10th Street Larue Carter Hospital building in Indianapolis.

The gap in information about INPA between 1942 and 1947 was not easy to fill. Dr. Reed recalled informal meetings in the homes of various Indianapolis psychiatrists during WWII but recalled no scientific papers, "just social gatherings to keep the spirit of the psychiatric group alive." It is likely that formal meetings were held in 1945-46 but those minutes did not survive.

During WWII public interest in psychiatry grew by leaps and bounds because of the public's exposure to "war neurosis," now know as post traumatic stress disorder. INPA set up a series of public seminars in the Indianapolis Shortridge High School Auditorium in which INPA members, psychologists and clergy participated. Panel discussions on mental health were held and INPA's second President, Dr. E. Vernon Hahn, was very active in these meetings which went on for at least two years. Dr. Hahn was a neurosurgeon who had studied analysis at Chicago and was generally regarded as "exceedingly brilliant and a good speaker."

E. Vernon Hahn served again as INPA president from January 1947 to October 1949. Dr. Reed described him as "a very well-organized person who readily accepted the scientific discipline from his earliest years." He set the post WWII example for many of the officers that followed in arranging for papers well in advance and having as many speakers as possible from out of state and elevating the tone of the psychiatric association to a fairly high scientific level.

Other early INPA Presidents were a varied lot: Dr. E. Rogers Smith (1940) was a private practitioner, primarily in neurology, after a number of years on the faculty at Indiana University School of Medicine. Neuropsychiatrist L. H. "Toby" Gilman, M.D., (1941) died while in office. He was known for his reticence to reveal his real first name, which was Harry. Dr. Gilman's term was completed by Dr. Breutsch, a "fine German pathologist" at Central State Hospital who had earlier worked out the mechanism by which malaria helped paresis. Thus, during WWII, INPA found itself headed by a man who had served Germany aboard a submarine during WWI. In addition to chairing the Department of Psychiatry, teaching neurology and psychiatry at Indiana University School of Medicine, covering the psychiatric service at Indianapolis City Hospital and seeing "charity cases," David Boyd, M.D., managed to find time to serve as INPA President in 1942.

Much of the political activity of INPA in the 1940s centered on the drive to build an adequate number of state psychiatric hospitals. Phil Reed described INPA as "sporadically active politically." When it was felt that we badly needed added beds in the state mental hospital system, we became active. "As usual, organizations do not act as monoliths, but you have four or five people who are movers and six or eight people who will help them move."

Larue Carter, M.D. was one of the movers behind the undertaking to build new state hospitals but he had no idea that one of the hospitals would be named after him. He died in 1946, three years before the groundbreaking of the Indianapolis facility that would bear his name.

## War and New Hospitals

The most powerful advocate for improvement of the state mental health picture was not a psychiatrist at all, but a dermatologist, Norman Beatty, M.D., who was a good friend of Larue Carter. The son-in-law of former Indiana Governor Edward Jackson, Dr. Beatty was well-connected in the political community. He maintained a life-long interest in mental health treatment in Indiana and served for many years on the Indiana Mental Health Council, a group charged with upgrading state mental health care. Immediately after WWII this group decided that the backwardness of Indiana's facilities called for a catalyst to generate change. The interest in psychiatry generated by WWII had led to the rapid creation of residencies to provide formal psychiatric training for physicians. A model hospital was needed to train relatively large numbers of residents who would hopefully filter out into the state system and improve care.

Norman Beatty regularly attended INPA meetings to get a feel for what the psychiatrists in the state wanted and needed. INPA left it up to him to do the lobbying and he was a very powerful one-person lobby. Much of the planning for Beatty and Carter Hospitals took place during the years for which INPA has no records. Most of the strategy meetings took place at the Indianapolis home of Larue Carter, a small gray cottage at 4280 N. Meridian Street. There, Drs. Larue Carter, Norman Beatty, Earl Mericle, Phil Reed and a few others decided who would seek out which public officials and what the next move would be to convince the legislature to fund the hospitals.

All the actual work in the legislature was done by Dr. Beatty who possessed some of his father-in-law's political skills. He button-holed numerous legislators in the corridors of the Capitol Building and "didn't twist wrists, but certainly tweaked the cortices." The persistence of Beatty and this small group of determined INPA psychiatrists paid off. While in Robert Long Hospital just after the myocardial infarction that would soon claim his life, Dr. Beatty reported to Dr. Reed that he had just learned in a phone conference with the Indiana Mental Health Commission that the new hospital would be named after Larue Carter. Dr. Beatty died seventy-two hours later, not knowing that the second hospital would be named after him.

Dr. Reed, who was adopted by Ann Gant Carter after Larue Carter's death in January 1946, attended the 1949 ceremony during which the cornerstone of Larue Carter Hospital was laid. Carter and Indiana's Governor Henry Schricker were also among the dignitaries present. As planned, the hospital's focus was on residency training and it boasted fifteen residents in its first several years of operation under the direction of Superintendent Juul Nielsen.

During the late 1940s, INPA met seven times a year, not meeting in the summer or in December, a tradition which continues to this day. The attendance in the immediate post-war years was fifteen to forty. Attendances of forty resulted from the establishment of Larue Carter Hospital when Norways still had seven residents.

## Getting Started Again: INPA in the Early 50s[3]

INPA formally re-organized sometime in 1947, probably in the early months when an extended meeting was held at the Indianapolis Athletic Club. The beginnings of the re-organization were apparently humble. No one remembered to bill the members for dinners or to reimburse Dr. Hepburn who, two years later, finally asked the treasury for reimbursement. When Secretary Dwight Schuster wrote to the six INPA directors to ask permission for such reimbursement, the eminent E. Vernon Hahn, M.D., replied that he was unaware of even being a director of "our famous organization." In 1949

INPA's other directors included Drs. E. Rogers Smith, Louis Nie, C. Basil Fausset, Earl W. Mericle, and John Hare. They filled the role that Councilors now have in the Indiana Psychiatric Society.

In 1949 INPA Secretary-Treasurer Phil Reed resigned because of illness and Dwight Schuster was appointed to fill this office. Dr. Schuster served many years as INPA Secretary and kept every scrap of INPA correspondence that crossed his desk. We owe him an incredible debt, for he gave us the archives from which much of this history is taken, archives that bring alive the spirit and toil of a talented and industrious group.

## Four Dollar Steaks at the Athenaeum

From 1949 through the mid 1950s most meetings were held at the Athenaeum in Indianapolis and boasted a 6:00 PM social hour, followed by dinner, then business and scientific sessions. Four dollar sirloin steak dinners were the usual fare. Meetings were held monthly from September to June, excluding December, and attendance was generally around thirty to thirty-five members and a few guests. Meeting announcements went out by post-card.

The Marion Veterans Administration Hospital hosted INPA every October and the society arranged special meetings to hear speakers at Riley Hospital's Doctor's Dining Room. Efforts were made to schedule meetings in conjunction with ISMA and the Central Neuropsychiatric Association meetings. Meetings were also held at some unusual places such as the Indianapolis Naval Armory and the Superintendent's quarters at Larue Carter Hospital.

A purely social June meeting was always held at Dr. Hahn's farm at Eagle Creek in Indianapolis. Maps indicate that this large and delightful "playground" was probably inundated when the Eagle Creek Reservoir was built. These were light-hearted affairs that lasted "until exhaustion sets in" and featured "hiking, fishing, horseshoes, wood-chopping and milking if you wanted milk." The June 1955 meeting even featured square dancing with entertainment by the "Clermont Hot Shots." Clearly, this was a society that knew how to have fun.

## The Roots of Modern Practice

Scientific programs covered a gamut of neurologic, psychiatric and neurosurgical topics but also addressed political concerns. Speakers were usually members of INPA but nationally known speakers and American

Psychiatric Association officials were invited if they were in the area. Most frequently, two or three INPA members would form a panel or present short papers that would be followed by lively discussion. Neurology and psychiatry residents were responsible for programs from time to time and case presentations abounded. Efforts were made to rotate monthly topics among the three specialties but sometimes topics such as psychodynamics and reflexes in the distal stump of a patient with a transected spinal cord ended up on the same night (February 1950).

A look at the topics presented and membership reactions to them is most revealing. Facts which we now take for granted, such as neuropsychological testing or uses for electroconvulsive therapy, were new findings that generated excitement and discussion. Now obscure treatments such as electronarcosis, electrostimulation and pre-frontal lobotomy were discussed along with problems we no longer face, such as the treatment of "the neuropsychiatric tuberculous patient." The etiology of schizophrenia and other classic debates were aired. INPA sometimes planned meeting topics only one or two months in advance but they were not short on creativity; in April 1950 their meeting was a play, "Susan Comes to the Child Guidance Clinic."

Political topics were less frequently found on the meeting agenda, but represented some of the "hotter" topics. A good example of this is the November 1949 meeting where a panel discussed coordinating INPA, the Indiana Mental Hygiene Society, and the Mental Health Council of Indiana. This meeting featured the report of the INPA liaison committee to the Indiana Mental Health Council and was attended by Indiana Governor Henry Schricker. The INPA report was critical of low salaries for state hospital doctors, the failure of the administration to abolish political appointments to state hospital jobs, and lack of funding to "staff the psychiatric institutions with attendants of the cultural level required for decent care of the mentally ill." The Governor was understandably less than enthused about the report and responded by pointing out the "financially embarrassed" situation of the state. It was not a boring meeting by any stretch of the imagination.

The paranoia of the McCarthy era is also evident in the archives. The March 1950 meeting featured observations on socialism in England; in November 1950 civil defense for the atom bomb was discussed. An October 1951 meeting on future programs for the care and treatment of veterans drew comments that the ideas of the Veterans' Administration Hospital speaker, Dr. Harvey Tompkins, were "definitely socialistic."

## A Tight-Knit Little Group

In 1949 INPA had fifty-two members led by three officers and six "directors" but this structure was anything but static. As INPA grew, numerous revisions of its societal structure occurred. In March 1949 the membership list and procedures were revised so that membership would only be granted after written application and investigation of the individual's qualifications. This revision came in response to difficulties in establishing the credentials of physicians who emigrated from war-torn Europe. By July of 1952 a membership committee existed and membership in the local medical society was necessary for active membership in INPA.

No copy of the old INPA constitution exists and its contents can only be inferred from the functioning of the society from 1947-50. In 1950 INPA restructured its council and seven councilors were elected to terms of one through seven years. Each year thereafter one councilor was to be replaced by a new councilor who would then serve a seven-year term. The next five years brought a confusing succession of structural changes.

Prior to 1952 presidents had been elected for one year and took office around October. In April 1952, the Council announced a slate of candidates that would take office the following October and serve two years "as outlined by the INPA constitution." Biennial elections were to take place in May of even-numbered years. In October 1952 Dr. E. Rogers Smith became the first president under this revised but very short-lived system.

In February 1954 a constitutional amendment was drafted to change officer's tenure to one year on a January to December basis. Parts of the proposed constitutional amendment were referred back to the council by a membership that was interested in a smaller council with more flexibility than offered by seven-year councilor terms offered. The final amendment proposed three officers to be elected annually and three councilors who would serve two-year terms and then would be ineligible to serve for one year. All seven of the current councilor positions were to be vacated by the first election which was held in October 1954. Thereafter, annual elections were to occur in November. Dr. H.C. Dunstone was elected president and served 1954 until December 1955 as this new system was put in place.

The functioning of the council was much more informal than today and reflected the close personal ties among the officers, a group of about ten males whose names appear again and again in various offices and committees. In November 1951 when Dr. Hahn announced that E. Rogers

Smith was in Florida convalescing from tuberculosis, the council promptly voted to send him a case of his favorite whiskey with INPA's best wishes. Dr. Smith wrote that this "was the best use of treasury funds ever made" by "the Lodge known as INPA," and inquired if they were trying to change his diagnosis from granuloma to delirium tremens!

In 1952 the dues were twelve dollars for active members, seven dollars for associate members. Residents had no dues but lacked voting privileges. For many years two dollars of the annual INPA dues were given to the Indiana Association for Mental Health for support of its activities, particularly lobbying. This was eliminated during a February 1954, dropping dues to ten dollars yearly.

In August 1950 INPA boasted fifty-three members, two honorary members, six associate members and nine residents. In 1952 residents were placed on the mailing list and offered dues-free membership. By 1953, INPA had grown to sixty regular members and twenty-five residents. INPA members were encouraged to host residents at meetings as a way of furthering the growth of the society.

## Relationship with the American Psychiatric Association

In August 1947 Dr. David Boyd sent the constitution and bylaws to the American Psychiatric Association as part of an application for affiliate status. This correspondence was misfiled by the American Psychiatric Association so affiliate status was not granted until after June 1948. The committee chairs of INPA communicated with corresponding sections in the American Psychiatric Association and sent news items to the American Psychiatric Association newsletter. In August 1950 the relationship between American Psychiatric Association district branches and affiliate societies was raised by a member of the American Psychiatric Association Council. At the October INPA meeting the issue of remaining an affiliate versus becoming a district branch was debated at length. Drs. E. Vernon Hahn, John Greist and Murray DeArmond were appointed to study the matter. Ten days later they recommended going for American Psychiatric Association district branch status. This would mean changing the INPA constitution so that all members were American Psychiatric Association members. Becoming a district branch meant having a larger voice in the policies of the American Psychiatric Association, a move which the American Psychiatric Association found desirable as it pushed for "furthering the democratic plan" by decentralizing its power. INPA Councilors were divided about the desirability of district branch status. Apparently several years of discussion took place in the American Psychiatric Association between 1950 and 1952 about whether district branches were to be favored over affiliate societies. In July 1952 the American Psychiatric Association issued a statement assuring each group that they were equally valued. Affiliate societies such as INPA often had neurologist and neurosurgeons as members. In 1953 INPA had twenty-two members who were not American Psychiatric Association members and some of these were psychiatrists.

In August 1953 the American Psychiatric Association wrote to Indiana about a study it was conducting to give more recognition and benefits to affiliate societies. INPA was not yet a district branch. On February 10, 1954 Dr. John Greist moved that district branch qualifications be complied with and INPA apply for district branch status in the American Psychiatric Association. This passed the council and the petition is dated February 26. This meant that INPA would no longer exist as an affiliate society. The next president, Dr. C. Keith Hepburn, was chosen because INPA wanted a president who would be eligible for American Psychiatric Association fellowship. On April 14, 1954 at a meeting held at the Naval Armory in Indianapolis, the INPA council announced the approval of INPA's request for American Psychiatric Association district branch status. On May 3, 1954 the American Psychiatric Association Assembly, meeting in St. Louis, approved the establishment of the Indiana District Branch. Dwight Schuster was appointed as delegate to the assembly in June 1954. Representation in the Assembly was one vote per twenty APA members and INPA had fifty-seven members who were American Psychiatric Association members.

Today the Indiana Psychiatric Society continues much as it did in the 1950s. Monthly scientific meetings continue to be held except during December and the summer months. The Indiana Psychiatric Society council is considerably enlarged, however, and contains the president, president-elect, secretary, treasurer, assembly representative and deputy representative, legislative representative, public affairs representative, and two counselors. There are many committees including continuing medical education, child, disaster, fellowship, diversity, ethics, geriatric, membership, private practice, and nominating. Now both fall and spring continuing medical education meetings are held. The current recession and loss of pharmaceutical company support has dented the budget, however, and dues are considerably more than twelve dollars a year now.

## Northern Indiana Psychiatric Society[1]

The Northern Indiana Psychiatric Society was conceived on November 20, 1957 at a meeting at the St. Joseph County Guidance Clinic in South Bend, Indiana. It arose out of the desire of the psychiatric staff at Norman Beatty Hospital in Westville to form a professional society of psychiatrists in the northwest corner of Indiana. This initial meeting was attended by twelve physicians. Over the next several months more meetings were held and a constitution and bylaws were written, modeled after the Indiana Neuropsychiatric Association constitution. A small group of psychiatrists, presumably all men, called for a "surrender of biases and enlargement of the field of one's clinical vision" to come together, share, inform, and enlighten one another and "to become as one man in the practice of psychiatry in northern Indiana." The Northern Indiana Psychiatric Society encompassed the seventeen counties in the northwest corner of the state, which was, at the time, the catchment area of Norman Beatty Hospital.

The psychiatrists who initially founded the Northern Indiana Psychiatric Society worked in a variety of settings including the Indiana State Prison, Norman Beatty Hospital, and private practice. At their monthly meetings they discussed case reports, forensic medicine, and other psychiatry-related topics. They hoped to develop a liaison with those in other professions including the law, ministry, social service, and politics.

The first official meeting of the Northern Indiana Psychiatric Society was on April 23, 1958 with Dr. Grant E. Metcalf presiding as president. By May 1958 the fledgling organization became a district branch of the American Psychiatric Association. There were nineteen charter members and by 1965 the membership reached thirty-one. The group held monthly meetings except during the summer and published a monthly newsletter.

## Mental Health of America in Indiana

In April 1915 the Indiana Board of State Charities requested the governor form a committee of eight individuals to study the plight of the feebleminded, epileptic, and insane. Committee members included George Edenharter, M.D., superintendent of Central State Hospital, Samuel Smith, M.D., superintendent of Richmond State Hospital, Charles Emerson, M.D., from Indiana University School of Medicine, Walter VanNuys, M.D., superintendent of the Indiana Village for Epileptics at New Castle, George Bliss, superintendent of the School for Feebleminded at Fort Wayne, Senator Frank Culbertson of Vincennes, and Representative Frank

Garvish, chairman of the State Board of Charities. In 1916 this group held an Indiana Conference on Mental Defectives. The well-known Clifford Beers, author of *A Mind that Found Itself,* spoke at this meeting. At this conference the Indiana Committee for Mental Hygiene was formed and this group eventually became the Indiana Mental Health Association.[1]

In its early years the Indiana Committee for Mental Hygiene was involved in the education of the general public about mental illness. The organization was inactive between 1936 and 1939 and during WWII ceased to function at all. After the war, when the body was resurrected, it was called the Indiana Society for Mental Hygiene. The society was partly responsible for forming the Indiana Council for Mental Health, the state agency responsible for state hospital system. In 1949 Marion County became the first local chapter. From 1950 to 1957 such notable psychiatrists as Drs. Murray DeArmond, Philip Reed, John Greist, Louis Nie, and DeWitt Brown served as chairpersons of the board. From 1953 to 1957 fifty-three new county chapters were formed. During the mid to late 1950s the Mental Health Association heavily lobbied the Indiana Legislature for more funds for mental health. Over the intervening years the Indiana Mental Health Association has continued to exert a strong voice in government and has lobbied for the formation of community mental health centers, the creation of the Institute of Psychiatric Research at Indiana University School of Medicine, and insurance parity on mental health.

This association is now called Mental Health of America in Indiana, an affiliate of the national organization. Currently Indiana has sixty local chapters.

## Conclusion

Organized psychiatry and mental health advocacy have come a long way in size, organization and advocacy since their early beginnings on the porch of the French Lick Springs Hotel. We owe much to the founders of INPA (now the Indiana Psychiatric Society) and to Drs. Philip Reed and John Greist, Sr., who provided interviews and recollections for the 1980 articles in the *Indiana Psychiatric Society Newsletter* that formed the basis for much of this chapter. Sadly, both of these gentlemen have now passed on to the next life.

## CHAPTER 10

# Department of Psychiatry, Indiana University School of Medicine

"A magician pulls rabbits out of hats. An experimental psychologist pulls habits out of rats."

Anonymous

## Introduction[1-2]

Prior to 1939 Indiana University School of Medicine had no full-time instructors in psychiatry. On July 1, 1939 David Boyd, M.D., became the first full-time instructor in psychiatry and in 1940 he was appointed the first official chair of the newly formed Department of Psychiatry, which was a part of the Neuro-Psychiatry Department. Other early clinical instructors in psychiatry prior to 1940 included Philip Reed, M.D., Earl Mericle, M.D., John Greist, Sr., M.D., and Keith Hepburn, M.D. With the help of Louis Nie, M.D., a course was developed for junior medical students at Indiana University School of Medicine. Under Dr. Boyd's leadership a psychiatry resident rotation was organized at Indianapolis City Hospital and Norways Hospital. The sophomore medical student course in psychopathology began in 1947.

Around 1949 Dr. Boyd accepted a position at the Mayo Clinic and Dr. Herbert Gaskill, M.D., from Philadelphia became the department chair. Under his leadership the department became much more academically and psychoanalytically oriented. A psychosomatic study group was formed in collaboration with the Chicago Psychoanalytic Institute. In 1952 the Neuro-Psychiatry Department at Indiana University School of Medicine was formally separated into two departments, Psychiatry and Neurology.

When Dr. Gaskill left in 1953, Alexander Ross, M.D., chair of the Department of Neurology became interim chair of the Department of

Psychiatry. Unfortunately, with the departure of Dr. Gaskill as chairman in 1953 and Dr. Juul Nielsen as superintendent of Carter Hospital in 1955, there was a decline in both the Psychiatry Department and its residency training program. From July of 1955 until July of 1956, only one of four newly appointed psychiatry residents stayed with the program. The number of psychiatric physicians at Carter Hospital declined to only two.

Better days arrived, however, in 1956 when John I. Nurnberger, Sr., M.D., from the Institute of Living and Yale University Hartford, Connecticut, was recruited as the Psychiatry Department chair. All eight residents who began their residency in 1957 stayed with the program. With the arrival of Dr. Nurnberger a remarkable period of growth began in the department. The Institute of Psychiatric Research became fully operational. Edward Tyler, M.D., was recruited as director of the Riley Child Psychiatry Clinic and Marion DeMyer, M.D., was recruited to run the childhood autism research unit at Carter Hospital. When Dr. Nurnberger retired in 1974 Hugh Hendrie, M.B., Ch.B., became chair of the Department of Psychiatry.

### Indiana University School of Medicine
### Department of Psychiatry Chairs:

| | |
|---|---|
| David A. Boyd, Jr., M.D. | 1939-1949 |
| Herbert S. Gaskill, M.D. | 1949-1953 |
| Alexander T. Ross, M.D., (Acting) | 1953-1956 |
| John Nurnberger, Sr., M.D. | 1956-1974 |
| Hugh C. Hendrie, M.B., Ch.B. | 1974-2001 |
| Christopher J. McDougle | 2001 |

What follows are historical descriptions of some of the special training programs and psychiatric facilities in the Department of Psychiatry at Indiana University School of Medicine.

## Training Programs

### Residency Training Program

In 1937 a one-year residency in neuropsychiatry was offered at Indianapolis City Hospital. In 1938 it was changed to a one-year residency in psychiatry and then to a two-year residency in 1939. The residency was first approved for three years in 1945. Some of the first-year residents in psychiatry were Louis Nie, M.D., in 1939, DeWitt Brown, M.D., in 1946, George Weinland in 1948, and Marilyn Caldwell, M.D., in 1949.[1]

By 1960 the residency training program at Indiana University School of Medicine had matured. Residency placements were available at Larue Carter Hospital, Marion County General Hospital, Veterans Administration Hospital, Long Hospital Adult Psychiatry Clinic, and Riley Hospital Child Guidance Clinic. The first full year was provided at Carter Hospital with six months on the male patient service and six months on the female patient service. During the second and third years residents spent three months on neurology, three months at Marion County General Hospital, six months in the Long Hospital Adult Psychiatry Clinic, six months at the Riley Hospital Child Guidance Clinic, and six months on an elective. Resident didactics included material on clinical syndromes, interview technique, personality development, psychological testing, psychotherapy techniques, forensic psychiatry, psychoanalytic theory, and the diagnosis and treatment of children. A resident journal club was held. Other regular educational conferences included inpatient team meetings and case conferences. Residents were expected to attend Saturday morning didactic sessions in the Neurology Department when they were on the neurology rotation. During their six months of elective time, psychiatry residents could spend time at any of the other state hospitals, the state facilities for the mentally retarded at Fort Wayne and Butlerville, and the state epilepsy hospital at New Castle. A two-year child fellowship was offered and residents could be boarded in the newly developed subspecialty of child psychiatry. The training in child psychiatry included consultation with pediatrics, schools, courts, and residential treatment facilities. Rotations for child fellows occurred at Riley Child Guidance Clinic, Riley Pediatric Clinic, Larue Carter Hospital Inpatient Children's Service, and the Marion County Child Guidance Clinic. Yearly resident stipends in 1960 were $4,854 for first year, $5,400 for second year, $6,800 for third year, $6,900 for fourth year, and $7,800 for fifth year.[2]

The earliest available composite photograph of the psychiatry residents in the 1964-65 year shows these residents: Drs. W. Winston Barnard, J. Kenneth Cooke, David G. Crane, William H. Davis, William P. Egan, Joseph P. Ficable, Sherman G. Franz, Roger K. Hinesley, Philip J. Holmes, Howard M. Luginbill, Ned P. Masbaum, Philip M. Morton, Noreen M. O'Connell, Nicholas Pappas, Jerry M. Ross, Clyde B. Rountree, Takuya Sato, Robert E. Snodgrass, George A. Teabolt, Jean A. Warren, and John

Y. Yarling. In the 1965-66 year Drs. H. Lane Ferree, Lowell Foster, Mary Murphy, Robert Snodgrass, Frank Walker, and James Wright were newly pictured faces. In the 1967-1968 year new faces included Drs. Gloria Bixler, Judith Edwards, John Henderson, Leonard Lawrence, Jon Leipold, William Shriner, Paul Stewart, Barbara Stillwell, and David Whelage. Drs. Fred Buehl and Larry Davis appeared in the 1968-69 year. These psychiatry residents went on to become faculty members in the Department of Psychiatry, physicians in community mental health centers, and Indiana private practitioners of psychiatry.[3] It is gratifying to see the change over the years from a virtually all Caucasian male psychiatry residency to a multinational residency group which is composed of nearly equal numbers of male and female residents.

Over the years the Indiana University School of Medicine psychiatry residency training program has educated numerous psychiatrists who spread all over Indiana as well as many other states. Some of the early trainees practiced in Bloomington (David Crane), Columbus (Sherman Franz and Jon Holdred), Fort Wayne (Joseph Ficable and Richard Mann), Mishawaka, Muncie (John Yarling), (Jon Leipold), Paoli (Wallace Shellenberger), South Bend (David Wehlage), Terre Haute (Lowell E. Becker and William Shriner), and Vincennes (John Henderson and James Koontz).

Chairpersons of the Residency Training Committee and Directors of the Psychiatry Residency Training Program from the early 1960s include the following:

| | |
|---|---|
| John Kooiker, M.D. | -1974 |
| Franklin Walker, M.D. | 1974-1979 |
| Clare Assue, M.D. | 1979-1990 |
| John Vara, M.D., & Roger Jackson, M.D. | 1990-1995 |
| Mary Landy, M.D. | 1995-1998 |
| Alan Schmetzer, M.D. | 1998-2010 |

## Medical Student Education in Psychiatry

Drastic changes have occurred in the training of medical students in psychiatry over the years. Medical students originally had psychiatry lectures in the Pathology Building at Central State Hospital. In the late 1960s there existed a series of lectures about the basic neurosciences in the freshman year. This course was based on the book *An Introduction to the Science of Human Behavior* by John I. Nurnberger, Sr., M.D. In the sophomore year medical students participated in a psychiatry course based on the book edited by Drs. Nancy Roeske and Clare Assue, *Examination of the Personality*. This new course was part of the medical school's newly revamped course called the Introduction to Medicine. The junior year consisted of a four-week psychiatric rotation at Larue Carter Hospital, University Hospital, Riley Hospital, Veterans Hospital, or General Hospital. Senior electives in psychiatry were available not only at Indiana University School of Medicine but throughout the state.

Currently freshman medical students have a twenty-week series of small group discussions in the Introduction to Clinical Medicine I. These discussions, which are co-led by a primary care physician and a psychiatrist are designed to bridge the gap between the basic and clinical sciences by focusing on medical ethics and the doctor-patient relationship. Sophomore medical students participate in the Introduction to Clinical Medicine II course. The psychiatric section of this course consists of a series of thirteen lectures given by psychiatrists. About half of the lectures are followed by interviews of volunteer psychiatric patients chosen to demonstrate various clinical syndromes. After the lectures, students meet in small discussion groups led by psychiatrists. The third year consists of a traditional one-month psychiatric clerkship at one of the numerous psychiatric facilities at Indiana University School of Medicine. A much greater emphasis is placed now on outpatient treatment and preparation of what a medical generalist should know. In addition, an emphasis is placed on training the medical student to master various clinical competencies in psychiatry. Psychiatric electives can be taken in the senior year as in the past.

## Section of Psychology

In 1956 Eugene Levitt, Ph.D., was hired to head the Section of Psychology, which at the time had three other members. Over the next fifteen years the Section of Psychology grew to nine members, with six at Riley Child Psychiatry Clinic and three in adult psychiatry. Members of the Section of Psychology for the first twenty years included Drs. Aare Truumaa, Bernard Lubin, Clayton Ladd, Gerald Alpern, Jacqueline French, Charles Perkins, Richard Snider, Frank Connolly, George McAdoo, and Richard Lawlor.[1]

Larue Carter Hospital established an internship program in psychology in 1955 and Indiana University School of Medicine established their psychology internship in 1957. Both programs were accredited by the

American Psychological Association and later merged in 1979. At its peak, there were twelve psychology interns in the program, largely thanks to funding from the National Institute of Mental Health. Eventually training included not only the Riley, Carter, Wishard, and VA Hospital facilities, but St. Vincent's Stress Center and Gallahue Community Mental Health Center in Indianapolis. Program directors for the IU internship include Drs. Eugene Levitt (1957-70), Aare Truumaa (1970-75), George McAdoo (1975-80), Elgan Baker (1980-88), Richard Lawlor (1987-97), and Linn LaClave (1997-2009). Directors of the Larue Carter Hospital program were Drs. Peter Lewinsohn, George Siskind, Art Sterne, and Robert Ten Eyck.[1-2]

## Division of Social Service

The Indiana University Division of Social Service program was located in Indianapolis. Social service field placements were available at Carter Hospital, Riley Hospital Child Guidance Clinic, and the Long Hospital Adult Psychiatry Clinic, all on the Indiana University Medical Center Campus. In 1960 social service staff at Carter Hospital included Ruth Copeland, Grace Green, John Murray, Doris Rodman, Ruth Rogers, Theodore Alex, Edward Bell, Barbara Coleman, Genevieve De Hoyos, Wilbur Dougherty, Angela Eckstein, Richard Henning, Meredith Lukenbill, Jeannne Luna. Social Service staff at the Riley Child Guidance Clinic included Edith Beatty, Patricia Henshaw, Sue Bragiel, Mary Jane Covalt, Esther Jones, and Julia Joseph. At Marion County General Hospital were Juliana Dober and John Hannon. William Baker was at Long Hospital and Jacque Sneed served at Veterans Hospital.

### Psychiatric Facilities

## Institute of Psychiatric Research

The Institute of Psychiatric Research on the Indiana University School of Medicine campus was formally dedicated on December 3, 1956. The $1,500,000 four-story building was financed by the Division of Mental Health. Dignitaries on hand for the dedication included Governor George Craig, Commissioner of Mental Health Margaret Morgan, M.D., Daniel Blain, M.D., president of the American Psychiatric Association, Indiana University president Herman Wells, and Department of Psychiatry chair John Nurnberger, Sr., M.D. Money to run the institute was to come from both public and private funds funneled through a nonprofit organization. The hopes for the institute were to discover ways to prevent mental illness and shorten the length of treatment for those already diagnosed.[1]

A small group of researchers, the future occupants of Institute of Psychiatric Research, arrived on the Indiana University School of Medicine campus in the fall of 1955. However, the new building was not ready for occupation until the fall of 1957. By that time Morris Aprison, Ph.D., Harvard Armus, Ph.D., Arthur Drew, M.D., Hanus Grosz, M.D., Harold Persky, Ph.D., Marvin Zuckerman, Ph.D., and John Nurnberger, Sr., M.D., had been busy at work in temporary quarters on the Indiana University School of Medicine campus. Other consultants and research collaborators included Orville Bailey, M.D., Eugene Levitt, Ph.D., Marian DeMyer, M.D., William DeMyer, M.D., James Norton, M.A., and Edward Tyler, M.D. At the end of 1958 the Institute had six full-time scientists, four part-time scientists and administrators, one senior research fellow, and five clinical and scientific consultants in addition to a number of research assistants, secretaries, maintenance workers, and animal care staff.[2]

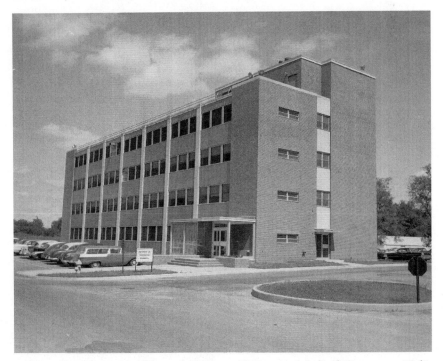

Institute of Psychiatric Research, Indiana University Medical Center, ca. 1960

By the end of the second year of official operation, the second annual report of the Institute of Psychiatric Research expressed the hope that the causes of various mental illnesses could be elucidated and that treatment could move from a trial and error approach to an approach with a more scientific backing. To realize these hopes interdisciplinary research groups were organized at the Institute. John Paul Brady, M.D., joined the Institute in July of 1959 and Harry Brittain was brought on board as a research assistant. A research ward at Larue Carter Hospital was started to study autistic children. Collaborators from various clinical departments of the Indiana University School of Medicine campus were engaged to participate in research efforts.[3]

After John Nurnberger, Sr., M.D., retired as director of the Institute in 1974, Morris Aprison, Ph.D., was appointed director. He stepped down in 1978 when John Nurnberger, Jr., M.D., became director.

Over the years the Institute has become a leader in psychiatric research, particularly in the areas of neurochemistry and neurobiology. When John Nurnberger, Jr., M.D., assumed the role of director a major thrust of research efforts was directed towards understanding the genetics of bipolar disorder. Other prominent research efforts have been on anxiety disorders, Alzheimer's disease, and the genetics of alcoholism.

## Larue D. Carter Memorial Hospital

This teaching and research state hospital was located on the campus of Indiana University School of Medicine until 1996 when it moved to the former Veterans Administration Hospital building several miles away on Cold Springs Road. See Chapter 4 for a description of the history of Larue D. Carter Memorial Hospital and the psychiatric teaching conducted there.

## Long Hospital Adult Psychiatry Clinic

The Long Hospital Adult Psychiatry Clinic was located in the "Cottages," a two-story former nursing residence hall located between Long and Coleman Hospitals on the Indiana University School of Medicine campus. At that time the staff consisted of three full-time psychiatrists, four psychiatric consultants, two psychologists, and one psychiatric social worker. Trainees included three psychiatry residents and two graduate social work students. The clinic offered both outpatient treatment and consultation to medical inpatients at Long Hospital, which was the then Indiana University adult general hospital. Most of the outpatients came from Marion County and its adjacent counties. The clinic population grew by about thirty-three percent between 1957 and 1960. As was usual in most outpatient psychiatric settings, women patients outnumbered men by about a third. Sixty-two percent of the patient population was between the ages of twenty-one to forty-four. Psychiatric diagnoses included personality disorders (thirty-one percent), psychoneuroses (twenty-seven percent), psychoses (twenty-one percent), brain syndromes (seven percent), psychophysiologic disorders (six percent), transient situation disturbances (three percent), and mental deficiency (one percent). About twenty-nine percent of patients initially seen for intake were treated at the clinic. The median number of treatment sessions was about eight but ranged from one to over one hundred.[1]

## Indiana University Hospital

Indiana University Hospital replaced Long Hospital on the Indiana University Medical Center campus. The hospital was built in phases, the first opening in 1970, a second a few years later, and the another in 1992. For many years the hospital had a psychiatric ward on the fourth floor and its longest serving director was Richard French, M.D. At one time this inpatient unit housed both adult and adolescent patients. After the formation of Clarian Health Partners in 1996 and the merger of Indiana University Hospital, Riley Hospital for Children, and Methodist Hospital, psychiatric inpatient services for both adults and adolescents were transferred to Methodist Hospital.

## Marion County General Hospital

Marion County General Hospital, formerly Indianapolis City Hospital, and later named Wishard Memorial Hospital, has always been a major training ground for psychiatry and has been a major provider of psychiatric treatment for indigent residents of Marion County.

Plans for the well-known medical/psychiatric detention unit at the hospital were actually formulated by the 1907 Indiana State Legislature. This unit was originally meant to be a holding place for those awaiting transportation to a state hospital as it was felt that a hospital setting was much better for these individuals than a county jail.[1]

In 1960 the psychiatry service had a forty-two-bed closed unit and a twenty-one-bed open unit. There were two outpatient clinics, one provided follow-up care after hospitalization and the other functioned as a teaching clinic with carefully selected outpatients. During the 1959-60 fiscal year 547 inpatients were admitted, sixty percent being admitted on a pre-mental examination warrant. In 1969 Indiana's first community mental health center, Midtown, opened and occupied the already existing psychiatric wards of General Hospital. See Chapter 8 for information about Midtown Community Mental Health Center.

## Riley Child Guidance Clinic

Until its name was changed to the Riley Child Psychiatry Clinic, the Riley Child Guidance Clinic was the child psychiatry clinic for Riley Hospital for Children on the campus of Indiana University School of Medicine. See Chapter 11 for details of this clinic's history and teaching programs.

## Veterans Administration Hospital

The Veterans Administration Hospital on West 10th Street, now know as Richard L. Roudebush Veterans Administration Medical Center, opened in 1952. Prior to the opening of the new hospital on West 10th Street, the main Veterans Hospital had been on Cold Springs Road, the current location of Larue Carter Hospital. In 1960 there were a total of seventy-eight inpatient psychiatric beds. During the 1959-60 fiscal year there were 338 admissions. Stuart Ginsberg, M.D., was the first director of the Psychiatry Department at the Veterans Hospital and he was followed by Hanus Grosz, M.D. In 1985 to 1995 Jack Sullivan, M.D., directed the Psychiatry Department. During his tenure Dr. Sullivan reorganized its services and accomplished considerable physical renovation of the Cold Springs Road psychiatric inpatient facilities. In the mid 1990s the Veterans Administration psychiatry service was relocated to the West 10th Street Veterans Hospital clearing the way for Larue Carter Hospital to move into the Cold Springs Road facility in 1996 in a land swap that provided more parking for Veterans Hospital employees at their West Tenth Street facility.

## Summary

Since 1975 the Psychiatry Department at Indiana University has undergone dramatic changes. Christopher McDougle, M.D., is the current chair. Groundbreaking basic science and clinical research continue at the Institute of Psychiatric Research and the various clinical facilities. With the opening of the Research II Building on the Indiana University Medical Center campus and its housing of the Paul and Carole Stark Neuroscience Research Institute, opportunities exist for expanded collaboration with the Departments of Neurology and Neurosurgery.

Currently the psychiatry residency training program for adult psychiatrists consists of four years. The first year has four months in primary care, two months in neurology, and six months on psychiatry inpatient services. The second year has a variety of rotations including geropsychiatry, forensic psychiatry, emergency psychiatry, addiction psychiatry, consultation liaison psychiatry, and child psychiatry. The third year consists of outpatient psychiatry and the fourth year is elective. Treatment of outpatients with long-term outpatient psychotherapy and continuous care with medication is built into the second through fourth years of the program. Joanna E. Chambers, M.D., is to become Director of Residency Training in late 2010.

Due to budgetary restraints, both the psychiatry residency and psychology internship programs are smaller. However, the psychiatry training program now offers training in two clinical tracks, clinical and academic/research. There is a triple-board program enabling residents to become boarded in adult psychiatry, child psychiatry and pediatrics. Fellowship experiences are offered in not only child psychiatry, but in geriatric psychiatry, addiction psychiatry, and psychopharmacology. The educational courses offered to psychiatry residents are being revamped.

## CHAPTER 11

# Child Psychiatry

"Grown-ups never understand anything for themselves, and it is tiresome for children to be always and forever explaining things to them."

Antoine de Saint-Exupery,
*The Little Prince,* 1943

Child psychiatry is a subspecialty of psychiatry which deals with the study, diagnosis, and treatment of psychiatric disorders occurring in childhood and adolescence. It is a relatively new twentieth-century discipline. Leo Kanner, M.D., (1894-1981), an Austrian psychiatrist, founded the world's first academic child psychiatry department at Johns Hopkins University in 1930. Kanner is considered to be the world's first child psychiatrist and his book, *Child Psychiatry,*[1] published in 1935, was the first English language child psychiatry text. One of Kanner's primary research interests was the study of childhood autism.

To become a child psychiatrist requires a physician to take three years of residency in general psychiatry and an additional two years in child psychiatry. Child psychiatry became the psychiatry's first subspecialty and its certification is available through the American Board of Psychiatry and Neurology.

We have chosen to discuss three representative child psychiatry clinics and hospitals in Indiana: the Riley Child Psychiatry Clinic, the Marion County Child Guidance Clinic, and the Evansville State Psychiatric Children's Center. More information about child psychiatry can be found in Chapter 4 under Larue Carter Memorial Hospital, Chapter 10 under residency training, and Chapter 13, which includes notable child psychiatrists such as Drs. Marion DeMyer, Helen Langner, Nancy Roeske, and James Simmons.

## Early Child Guidance Clinics at Indiana University School of Medicine

With the help of the Indianapolis Foundation, the first child guidance clinic in Indianapolis was established in 1927 in the basement of the Indiana University School of Medicine building. The clinic's director was Dr. Helen Langner who had a staff of two social workers and one psychologist. After two years the clinic folded because the university was forced to scale back expenses during the Great Depression.

In 1940 Herbert Cronick, M.D., who had been recruited by David Boyd, M.D., chair of the Department of Psychiatry, opened a new Child Guidance Clinic at the medical school. The clinic had two other employees, Mary Lee Cochran, a social worker, and Hazel Stevens, a psychologist. With the entry of the United States into World War II, however, Dr. Cronick soon left for the service and William Bowman, M.D., a psychiatry resident, filled in, but, within a year, he too left for the service. The clinic became inactive in 1942.[1]

## Riley Child Psychiatry Clinic[1-6]

The Riley Child Guidance Clinic at Riley Hospital for Children in Indianapolis, Indiana opened in the late 1949. At that time Marion County was behind other communities in both Indiana and the eastern United States in establishing child guidance clinics. Vanderburgh and Lake Counties in Indiana had previously established child clinics and Louisville, Kentucky had had a clinic since about 1925. Prior to 1947 the Riley Child Guidance Clinic was operated on a part-time basis by Hazel Stevens, Ph.D., Lillian Multon, M.D., and David Boyd, M.D. With the infusion of a seventy-five thousand dollar grant from the Indianapolis Junior League, the Indiana University School of Medicine was able to enlarge the clinic and open it full-time. Dr. John H. Waterman was its first full-time child psychiatrist director. In 1951 Samuel H. Warson, M.D., succeeded Dr. Waterman as clinic director. At that time plans were made to involve psychiatry residents in the clinic's operation. From 1954-56 Marilyn Caldwell, M.D., was clinic director.

When James Simmons, M.D., wrote about child psychiatry in Indiana in 1960, the Riley Child Guidance Clinic was still only one of twelve child guidance clinics in the state of Indiana. At the time Indiana was served by only one twenty-five-bed unit for children at Larue D. Carter Memorial Hospital. Other children and adolescents needing inpatient psychiatric treatment were housed on adult wards in other state mental hospitals. As of June 1959 these hospitals had 422 patients under age of eighteen on their rolls. Dr. Simmons made the following recommendations to the Indiana state legislature in 1960: 1) establishing a Section on Child Mental Health within the Division of Mental Health, 2) training of additional child psychiatrists, psychologists, social workers, and other staff for existing programs, 3) the building of three new residential treatment facilities, 4) the establishment of a research and training unit for children at Carter Hospital, 5) expansion of community child psychiatry clinics, and 6) additional financial support for existing child psychiatry clinics.

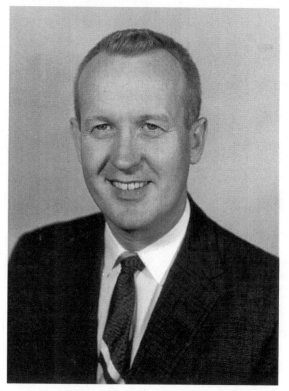

James E. Simmons, M.D.

After Dr. Simmons served as director of the Riley Child Guidance Clinic, other directors have included Drs. Nancy Roeske, Judith Campbell, Suzanne Blix, and David Dunn. The clinic was eventually renamed the Riley Child Psychiatry Clinic and was moved from its quarters in the oldest part of Riley Hospital to the new Riley Outpatient Center.

## Marion County Child Guidance Clinic[1-5]

The Marion County Child Guidance Clinic opened in late 1949 on East 11th Street in Indianapolis. Its first part-time director was Philip B. Reed, M.D. The building in which it was situated had two play therapy rooms and offices for psychiatrists, psychologists, social workers, and nurses. It also contained a library and auditorium. In 1953 Dr. James E. Simmons became clinic director and succeeded Dr. Alberta Jones, who had been clinic director for the previous two years. In 1961 Edward C. Shipley, M.D., a child psychiatrist, became clinic director. By that time the clinical staff had grown to seven social workers, two psychologists, and two psychiatrists. It was financially supported by the State of Indiana, United Fund, Indianapolis Public Schools, Marion County Juvenile Court, and the Public Welfare system. In 1978 the Marion County Child Guidance Clinic opened a second clinic, the Adult and Child Mental Health Center at 5145 Madison Avenue. This clinic eventually became a community mental health center that serves the southern part of Marion County and Johnson County.

## Evansville Children's Psychiatric Hospital

To meet the need for more inpatient beds for children in Indiana, the Evansville Psychiatric Children's Center was opened in 1966 five years after having been authorized by the Indiana State Legislature. Edward Tyler, M.D., a psychiatrist at Riley Child Guidance Clinic in Indianapolis, acted as a consultant for the planning of this hospital.[1] The hospital consisted of three buildings, one containing the school and administrative offices, the second containing patient housing, and the third containing recreation facilities. It served children from the ages of five to thirteen and currently has twenty-eight beds. One of dormitories served older boys and another served both younger girls and boys. Schooling was provided on site by the Evansville public school system. Currently there is one board-certified child psychiatrist on the staff and the hospital is accredited by the Joint Commission on Accreditation of Healthcare Organizations. The hospital has a full complement of treatment personnel including psychologist, social worker, nurses, recreational therapists, speech pathologist, dietary staff, and pediatrician.[1-3]

The first chief of the Evansville Psychiatric Children's Center was Charles L. Langsam, M.D. Prior to coming to Evansville Dr. Langsam had directed a children's psychiatric clinic in Long Beach, California after a seventeen-year child psychiatry experience in Cleveland, Ohio. Dr. Langsam did his medical training at Washington University in St. Louis and his residencies at Bellevue Hospital in New York and in Cleveland.[4]

Initially The Evansville Psychiatric Children's Center went through the usual growing pains of trying to attract qualified staff and fill beds. By its third year of operation the first two superintendents had resigned and in 1969 it had no psychiatrist on staff. Because of these problems, funds for operation were slashed and an interim study committee was appointed to study the situation.[5] In 1975 an Indiana legislative bill was proposed to allow private child psychiatrists to hospitalize their patients at the hospital.[6] In 2002 Governor Frank O'Bannon proposed closing the hospital as part of a state budget cutt.[7] However, the outcry against closing the hospital was so great that the Indiana Legislature passed a bill against closure.[8]

Currently Indiana continues to have both a shortage of child psychiatrists and inpatient beds for children and adolescents. One bright spot on the horizon is that there are plans for the Riley Hospital expansion to finally have a child psychiatry unit when completed in 2013.

# CHAPTER 12

# Notable Indiana Psychiatrists of the Nineteenth Century

"On Christmas Day – and nothing could befit the day better – the Superintendent invited a few friends and ordered a bonfire made of all the old instruments of restraint...The straps, halters, and cribs, were heaped together, making a pile twenty feet high. Then, in the presence of the rejoicing inmates and visitors, the torch was applied to the hideous pile, and the implements of restraint were consumed."

*Indianapolis Saturday Herald*, December 29, 1883 [as quoted in Rachael L. Drenovsky, Humanity's bonfire, William B. Fletcher, M.D., 1837-1907, *Traces*, Spring 2001, pp.18-25)

To become a psychiatrist in the nineteenth century required little beyond attending medical school and beginning work in one of the numerous hospitals for the insane which were established in the United States in the latter half of the century. What follows are vignettes of notable psychiatric physicians who worked in public and private psychiatric institutions in Indiana during the nineteenth and early twentieth centuries.

## James S. Athon[1-2]

Dr. Athon was born on April 11, 1811 in Louden County, Virginia. He received his medical degree from the Medical College in Louisville, Kentucky. He eventually settled in Charlestown, Indiana, and, when the Mexican War began, he was appointed surgeon of the Third Indiana Regiment. When he returned from the war he was elected to the Indiana State Senate.

From 1853-64 Dr. Athon was the third superintendent of the Indiana Hospital for the Insane (later to become Central State Hospital) in Indianapolis. As superintendent he introduced a precise method for recording physical and mental characteristics in the medical record.

In April 1857 the hospital's board of commissioners informed him that the Indiana General Assembly had failed to make appropriations for keeping the patients in the hospital. Subsequently Dr. Athon asked county clerks to remove their patients from the hospital. A total of 303 patients were discharged. The wards were reopened in October 1857 after the Indiana state treasurer assured the board that monies would be made available for the support of patients until the meeting of the next Indiana General Assembly in 1858.

In 1862 Dr. Athon was elected Secretary of State in Indiana. After his two-year term he resumed medical practice. He died on October 25, 1875.

### George Frederick Edenharter[1-5]

Dr. Edenharter was born on June 13, 1857 in Piqua, Ohio. Both of his parents had emigrated from Germany in 1848. In 1878 the family moved to Indianapolis where Edenharter worked in a cigar-making factory. He entered politics and ran for mayor in 1887 after having served on the Indianapolis City Council from 1884. Although he lost the mayoral race, his experience in government was quite helpful in his future career in hospital administration. He received his medical training at the Physio-Medical College of Indiana (1884) and the Medical College of Indiana (1886), both in Indianapolis. He was superintendent of City Hospital from 1889-93 and then became superintendent of Central State Hospital where he remained until he died in 1923. During his tenure at Central State Hospital Edenharter established a separate building on the grounds for the treatment of the criminally insane. He also had a series of lectures on forensic psychiatry for lawyers and law students. Endenharter was instrumental in the establishment of Madison State Hospital, the Indiana Village for Epileptics in New Castle, and the hospital for insane criminals within the Indiana State Prison at Michigan City. In 1908 Edenharter was chairman of the Indiana State Board of Charities and Corrections. He died on of a stroke in his residence on the grounds of Central State Hospital on December 6, 1923.

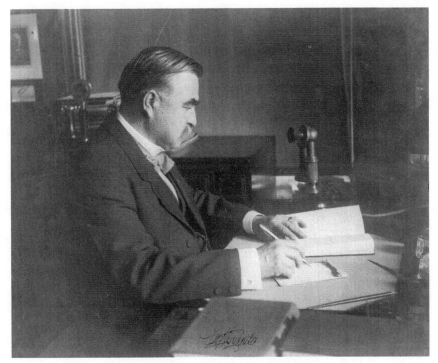

George Frederick Edenharter, M.D.

Though Dr. Edenharter's foresight, a pathology laboratory was built on the hospital grounds of Central State Hospital in 1895. Here lectures on neuro-pathology were offered to students from the Medical College of Indiana. In fact, the Pathology Building was the location of psychiatry teaching and research at Indiana University School of Medicine until Carter Hospital and the Institute of Psychiatric Research were established in the early 1950s. The old Pathology Building is now the Indiana Medical History Museum. Exhibits inside include a teaching amphitheatre, physician's and pathologist's offices, an autopsy room, three clinical laboratories (pathology, histology, and chemistry), a library, and an anatomical room containing numerous brain specimens. Outside is a medicinal plant garden.

## Orpheus Everts[1-4]

Dr. Everts was born on December 18, 1826 at the Salem Settlement in Union County, Indiana. He studied medicine with his father, Sylvanus Everts, M.D., and another physician, Daniel Meeker, M.D., in LaPorte,

Indiana. He obtained his medical degree in 1846 from Indiana Medical College in LaPorte, Indiana. After graduation he practiced medicine at St. Charles, Illinois. Subsequently he gave up the practice of medicine and became a newspaper editor in LaPorte, Indiana. He studied law and was admitted to the practice of law in 1860. During the Civil War he was a surgeon with the 20th Indiana Volunteer Infantry. He received honorary medical degrees from Michigan State University in 1865 and Rush Medical College in 1867. Subsequently he developed an interest in diseases of the nervous system and in 1866 he became superintendent of the Indiana Hospital for the Insane in Indianapolis where he remained for eleven years. During that time he was Chairman of the Department of Nervous and Mental Diseases at the Medical College of Indiana. In 1880 he became superintendent of the Cincinnati Sanitarium, a large private psychiatric hospital. In 1881 he was an expert witness in the trial of Charles Guiteau who assassinated President Garfield. From 1885-86 Dr. Everts was president of the Association of Medical Superintendents of American Institutions for the Insane, the forerunner of the American Psychiatric Association. Dr. Everts died on June 19, 1903 in Cincinnati, Ohio.

## William Baldwin Fletcher[1-5]

William Baldwin Fletcher, the son of Indianapolis banker and attorney, Calvin Fletcher, was born in Indianapolis on August 18, 1837. After attending private schools in Indianapolis and Indiana Asbury College (now DePauw University) in Greencastle, he graduated from the New York City College of Physicians and Surgeons in 1859. In 1861 at the onset of the Civil War, Dr. Fletcher enlisted in the Sixth Indiana Infantry, and, under the direction of John S. Bobbs, M.D., helped establish a hospital at Camp Morton in Indianapolis. While serving on detachment and under the command of General J.J. Reynolds, he was captured by the Confederates while on a scouting expedition in West Virginia. He was treated as a spy, sentenced to death, and narrowly escaped execution because of lost paperwork. In 1862 he was paroled as a prisoner of war and returned to Indiana. He married Agnes O'Brien in 1863 and established a partnership with Theophilus Parvin, M.D., who established the *Indiana Journal of Medicine* and published a major textbook on obstetrics. Until the close of the Civil War, Dr. Fletcher made travels to various battlefields to care for wounded soldiers. He also wrote letters to various Indianapolis newspapers and chided the city for its lack of attention to public safety and sanitation.

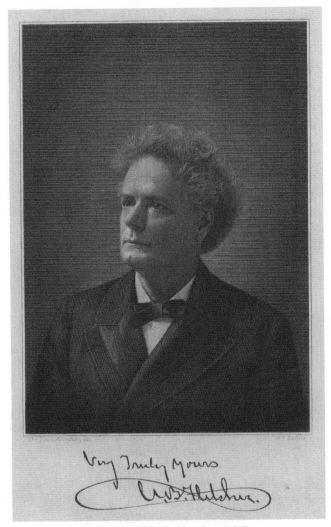

William Baldwin Fletcher, M.D.,
photo courtesy of Indiana Historical Society

In 1868 Dr. Fletcher helped organize Indiana Medical College where he eventually became chair of nervous and mental diseases. Later he helped establish the Central College of Physicians and Surgeons in Indiana where he also became chair of nervous and mental diseases. In 1870 he established the Indianapolis City Dispensary, a clinic for the city's disadvantaged poor and jailed prisoners. A Democrat, he was elected state senator from Marion County in 1882, and, during the time that he served a part term, he authored bills to improve public health and safety.

In June 1883 Dr. Fletcher agreed to become the superintendent of the Indiana Hospital for the Insane. Dr. Fletcher, always an innovator, hired Dr. Sarah Stockton, the hospital's first woman physician. He also appointed the first hospital chaplain, began patient dental care, and established a hospital school system. He abandoned secret burials on the hospital grounds and abolished medicinal alcohol (Three gallons per day had been consumed by the hospital.). It what must have been a spectacular show, he had all physical restraints burned in a large Christmas bonfire in 1883. This act was cheered by patients and hailed by many persons nationwide, although not by all hospital superintendents. He was fired in 1887 for exposing political corruption within his own hospital.

In 1888 Dr. William Fletcher opened the Fletcher Sanitorium, later known as Neuronhurst, the first private facility for the treatment of nervous and mental diseases in Indiana (See Chapter 5). Dr. Fletcher died on April 25, 1907 in Orlando, Florida.

## Joseph Goodwin Rogers[1-4]

Joseph Goodwin Rogers was born on November 23, 1841 in Madison, Indiana. In 1863 he studied medicine at the Cincinnati College of Medicine and subsequently obtained his medical degree from Bellevue Hospital Medical College in New York in 1884. During the Civil War he served as military surgeon at a military hospital near Madison, Indiana. From 1879-83 he was superintendent of Indiana Hospital for the Insane in Indianapolis. Subsequently he became medical engineer for the state of Indiana and presided over the construction of state hospitals at Richmond, Logansport, and Evansville. In 1888 he became superintendent of Logansport State Hospital. While at Logansport he named the hospital Longcliff because it was situated high on a bank overlooking the Wabash River.

Dr. Rogers was a frequent speaker before different medical societies and his papers were not always on nervous and mental diseases. For example, in 1874 shortly after graduation from college he read a paper before the American Railway Master Mechanic's Association on "Steam boiler incrustations, its causes, consequences, and prevention." He made a number of presentations about hospital construction. His other medical papers included "Carbolic acid in purulent ophthalmia," "Treatment of wounds of the eyeball," "Thyreoids in catalepsy," "First aids for the insane," "Cold as a cure for tetanus," and "Vocation in paretic dementia."

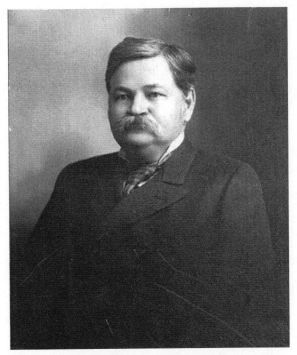

Joseph Goodwin Rogers, M.D.

Two of Dr. Rogers' papers are worthy of special note. The first, "The state and its insane," published in the *Indiana Bulletin of the Charities and Correction* in March 1899, gave an accounting of the number of "insane" persons enrolled in various facilities in Indiana. The state's mental hospitals held 3,336, county asylums contained 322, and county jails housed thirty-eight. Dr. Smith pegged the number of the state's insane at 4,300 or one in every 675 in population. Dr. Rogers was especially critical of the Indiana State Legislature which had failed to provide adequate space to house patients who had been judged insane.[5]

The second paper, "A century of hospital building for the insane," was a presidential address presented at the May 1900 Annual Meeting of the American Medico-Psychological Association. In his paper, Dr. Rogers noted the failure of the "Kirkbride Plan" of constructing psychiatric hospitals, which had resulted in hospital overcrowding on large poorly attended wards. Dr. Rogers suggested an alternative, the "Cottage Plan." The Cottage Plan consisted of a series of smaller buildings grouped around a common center, with each patient building housing twelve to twenty patients. Dr. Rogers described how each of these buildings should be constructed from the foundation upwards. Dr. Rogers also advocated that patients be grouped into different categories based upon their treatment needs. These groups included 1) "the noisy and violent, disturbed and disturbing," 2) "the quiet non-worker," 3) "the suicidal and epileptic," 4) "the quiet working class," 5) "the sick and infirm," and 6) "the neat, quiet, mutually agreeable class."[6]

From 1899 to 1900 Dr. Rogers was president of the American Medico-Psychological Association, forerunner of the American Psychiatric Association. Dr. Rogers died in Logansport, Indiana on April 11, 1908.

## Mary Angela Spink[1-3]

Mary Angela Spink, born November 18, 1863 in Washington, Indiana, was the daughter of a Daviess County druggist. She attended private schools, and, at the tender age of fifteen, shocked her community by announcing that she intended to become a physician. In order to pay for her medical education, she became a nurse. In 1882 she attended Pulte Medical College in Cincinnati, Ohio. In 1884 she returned to Indiana and became a special night nurse at the Indiana Hospital for the Insane in Indianapolis. From 1885 until 1887 she completed her medical studies at the Medical College of Indiana. She graduated with high honors and took a prize for dissection. In 1888 she took postgraduate courses in nervous and mental disease in New York. Following a year in private practice, she was hired by Dr. Fletcher as his assistant at Fletcher's Sanitarium or Neuronhurst. After three years she was made a partner and eventually became superintendent of the women's department. Following the death of Dr. Fletcher in 1907, she became superintendent of Neuronhurst. At her death in September 1937, Neuronhurst was still actively functioning, but closed shortly thereafter. During her career Dr. Spink was head of the Indiana Board of State Charities for thirty years. She devised a method to preserve "inter-cranial circulation." She served on the medical staffs of Indianapolis City Hospital and the Indianapolis City Dispensary. She belonged to a various professional societies and published a number of papers in the *American Journal of Microscopy* and the *Woman's Medical Journal*.

## Albert Eugene Sterne[1-2]

Dr. Sterne was born in Cincinnati, Ohio on April 28, 1866. Both of his parents had emigrated from Germany. He graduated from Harvard

University in 1887 and then obtained his M.D. degree at the University of Berlin in 1891. While in Europe he also studied in Austria, France, England, and Ireland. He came to Indianapolis in 1893 and was appointed chairman of the Department of Mental and Nervous Disorders at the Central College of Physicians in Indianapolis. In 1896 he established Norways Hospital. Dr. Sterne wrote many medical articles and was an associate editor of the *Journal of Nervous and Mental Diseases*. He died on June 30, 1931 in Denver Colorado where he had gone to visit his brother.

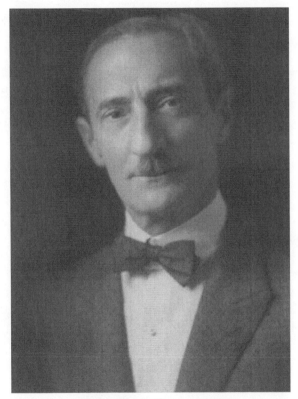

Albert Eugene Sterne, M.D.

## Sarah E. Stockton[1-3]

Dr. Stockton was born in Tippecanoe County, Indiana in 1842. She and her sister ran the Stockton Boarding House in Lafayette for some years. She obtained her M.D. degree in 1882 from the Woman's Medical College in Philadelphia, Pennsylvania. In December 1883 she came to the Indiana Hospital for the Insane in Indianapolis. She worked primarily on the women's wards for the next twenty-five years. While at the hospital she treated women's gynecological problems which were then thought to have at least partially caused insanity in women. At one point in her career she was Anna Agnew's physician (See Chapter 16). For a time Dr. Stockton worked at Fletcher's Sanitarium or Neuronhurst. Later she worked at both the Indiana Reform School for Girls and the Indiana Woman's Prison. Dr. Stockton died on the grounds of Central State Hospital on March 13, 1924 after her second hip fracture in two years.

### Andrew J. Thomas[1]

Dr. Thomas was born in Raymond, Mississippi on December 12, 1840. His undergraduate degree was from the University of Missouri. After the Civil War, which ruined his family financially, he graduated from Jefferson Medical College in Philadelphia in 1867. He started the practice of medicine in Oaktown, Indiana. For several years he was editor of the *Vincennes Sun*, but this venture failed. From 1879 to 1890 he was an assistant physician at the Indiana Hospital for the Insane in Indianapolis. In 1890 he became superintendent of the Southern Indiana Hospital for the Insane in Evansville. He retired from that position in 1897.

Although Dr. Thomas had moved North after the Civil War, he continued to have much fondness for his southern roots. With much glee, he later related an anecdote when he and several medical colleagues were passing by Governor's Circle (now known as Monument Circle) in Indianapolis after midnight, they made him kneel down in front of the statue of Oliver P. Morton (Indiana's Civil War governor) and renounce his "rebel sentiments." Dr. Thomas died on June 1, 1898.

## CHAPTER 13

# Notable Indiana Psychiatrists of the Twentieth Century

"Time wounds all heels" [Groucho Marx]

Sign on the desk of Donald F. Moore, M.D.,
superintendent of Larue D. Carter Memorial Hospital

The psychiatrists listed in this chapter by no means include all of the notable Indiana psychiatrists. Psychiatrists chosen for this chapter are notable from the respect that they influenced several generations of Indiana psychiatrists through their teaching efforts and their clinical, research, and administrative acumen. Most psychiatrists listed here are deceased and the few living ones mentioned are in their 80s or 90s. They deserve our enduring respect. They are listed here in alphabetical order. Newspaper articles, obituaries, and personal interviews, supplemented by the *Biographical Directory of the American Psychiatric Association*,[1] were primary sources of information for this chapter.

## Vincent Boone Alig

Dr. Vincent Alig graduated from Shortridge High School in Indianapolis in three years and then attended Purdue University where he began majoring in electrical engineering. After two years at Purdue he transferred to the University of Michigan at Ann Arbor where he obtained his bachelor's degree in psychology in 1948. In 1951 he completed his master's degree in psychology at Butler University. He obtained his M.D. degree from Indiana University School of Medicine in 1955. During an externship at Norways Hospital he performed psychological testing. He did a rotating internship at Indiana University School of Medicine and completed his psychiatry residency at the Menninger Clinic in Topeka, Kansas in 1959. After two years of service in the Army at Fort Monmouth, New Jersey, he began work as a staff psychiatrist at Larue Carter Memorial Hospital in 1961. For most of his psychiatric career Vince worked half-time as a treatment team supervisor at Carter Hospital and half-time in private practice at Methodist Hospital. In private practice he shared an office suite with Drs. John Kooiker, Frank Countryman, and Philip Reed.

In addition to performing psychological testing when he was at Norways, Vince observed insulin coma treatments. Vince recalled when he was a junior medical student, he and his classmates were introduced to hydrotherapy by the nursing staff at Carter Hospital and they actually had a hydrotherapy session, which he recalled as "very relaxing." Vince vividly recalled Alex Ross, M.D., giving neurology lectures and demonstrating various types of disordered gaits. Dr. Alig is retired from clinical practice.

## Clare Melba Assue[1-3]

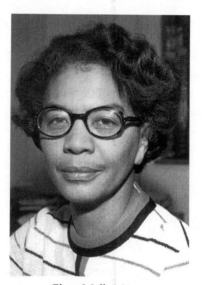

Clare Melba Assue

Dr. Clare Assue was a teaching legend at Larue Carter Memorial Hospital. Born on December 27, 1922 in New York City, she graduated from Hunter College in New York City in 1949 and received her M.D. degree from Howard University in Washington, D.C. in 1954. She interned at Beth-El Hospital in Brooklyn and completed her psychiatry residency training at St. Elizabeth's Hospital in Washington, D.C. after taking her first year of residency at Indiana University School of Medicine. She first came to Carter

Hospital in 1958. During her career at Carter Hospital she was chief of the Male Service for many years. Beloved by many psychiatric residents, she was a psychotherapy supervisor and headed the Psychiatry Residency Training Committee for many years. She was fond of telling the psychiatry residents that during World War II she worked as a welder in the Brooklyn Naval Yard. She was a real life "Rosie the Riveter." From 1981 until her retirement in 1989 she was superintendent of Carter Hospital. During her career in psychiatry she attained the rank of professor at Indiana University School of Medicine, served as coordinator of the Psychiatry Undergraduate Curriculum Committee, and was director of Medical Education at Carter Hospital. For many years she taught Interview Technique to first year psychiatry residents. She had a special gift for doing psychotherapy with schizophrenics who were amenable to this technique. She was a valued examiner for the American Board of Psychiatry and Neurology and received the prestigious Sagamore of the Wabash Award from Indiana's governor Robert Orr in 1987 for her public service. Not content with just her teaching role, she was active in many community organizations including the Parent Teachers Association at Shortridge High School, Board of Directors of St. Richard's School, Board of Directors of the Community Service Council, and member of the Juvenile Justice Commission. Dr. Assue died on August 28, 1990.

## Max A. Bahr[1-6]

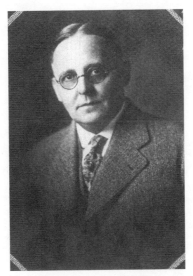

Max A. Bahr, M.D.

The son of Paul Bahr, pianist and composer, Dr. Bahr was born on March 21, 1872 in Indianapolis, Indiana. In 1896 he obtained his M.D. degree from the Central College of Physicians and Surgeons in Indianapolis. Following graduation he worked a year in the Indianapolis City Dispensary and then was chief resident physician of the Government Emergency Hospital in Washington, D.C. In 1899 he returned to Indianapolis as a physician at Central State Hospital. He took a leave of absence and obtained the degree of Doctor in Psychological Medicine from the University of Berlin in 1908.

After obtaining his advanced degree, Dr. Bahr returned to Central State Hospital. He was appointed superintendent in 1923 after the death of superintendent George Edenharter, M.D. During his tenure at Central Dr. Bahr established a course in forensic psychiatry for attorneys.[7] Under his leadership Central State Hospital became prominent in the malarial treatment of neurosyphilis. The hospital also introduced electroconvulsive therapy and insulin coma therapy while he was at Central. Dr. Bahr and Dr. Walter Bruetsch also studied the relationship of rheumatic fever to psychotic states or what eventually came to be termed rheumatic brain disease. While Dr. Bahr was at Central the patient population rose from fourteen hundred to twenty-three hundred after a number of new buildings had been erected, including a "sick hospital," three infirmaries, two general dining rooms, an amusement hall, and five cottages.

Dr. Bahr was a professor of psychiatry at Indiana University School of Medicine, whose medical students he routinely taught while he served at Central. Medical students attended his Saturday afternoon lectures in the amphitheater of the Pathology Building. He also offered psychiatric courses for student nurses and social workers.

Dr. Bahr consulted at the United States Federal Penitentiary in Terre Haute and also consulted with the Indianapolis Police and Fire Commission. He remained at Central until he retired in 1952.

Dr. Bahr published articles in a number of prominent psychiatric journals. He and Dr. Bruetsch published their experience with the malarial treatment of general paresis or late stage syphilis in the *American Journal of Psychiatry* in 1928.[8] Dr. Bahr also conducted studies on the relationship of rheumatic fever to psychoses. In *Modern Hospital* he published an early article about recreational and occupational therapy.[9] His interest in child psychiatry was apparent in the publication in the *Journal of the Indiana State Medical Association* of an article on psychiatric problems in children, in which he divided children's problems into neurotic, mentally defective, and psychotic categories. He urged the modern psychiatric evaluation of children in which complete developmental, family, personal, and educational histories were taken as well as the performance of a physical examination.[10] In child psychiatry he was far ahead of his time.

Upon his retirement, Dr. Bahr reflected on the field of psychiatry. He felt that when he started psychiatry, it was just emerging from its medieval period, thanks to Dorothea Dix and the reforms of the late nineteenth century. Psychiatric diagnosis was only in its infancy as there were only three diagnoses, "maniacal, melancholic, and demented." Human behavior was still a mystery. During Dr. Bahr's career the role of stress and personality was discovered. Physicians began to appreciate the mind-body interaction and psychosomatic illnesses. Electroconvulsive therapy and insulin coma therapy were introduced. Brain surgery to treat certain intractable mental illnesses became a reality. Psychoanalysis and psychotherapy were born. The novel idea of a psychiatric outpatient clinic arose. Finally, interest arose in the relationship of mental illness to crime.[11]

Besides being a top-notch scholar, Dr. Bahr had some interesting habits. He was a large man, weighing about two hundred forty pounds. He was used to starting his day with a hearty breakfast of bacon and eggs and then skimped on his remaining meals. Although he did not smoke, he chewed cigars. One wonders whether he acquired this particular habit from his colleague, Dr. George Edenharter, who began his career by making cigars. Dr. Bahr did not drink, although he had no problems with others who imbibed.

On January 24, 1953, after fifty-four years of service at Central State Hospital, Dr. Bahr died of a myocardial infarction at his home in Thorntown, Indiana.

# David A. Boyd, Jr.[1-3]

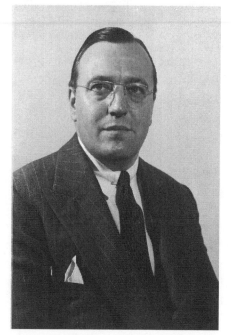

David A. Boyd, Jr., M.D.

Dr. Boyd was born in Detroit, Michigan. He received his undergraduate degree from the University of Michigan, his medical degree from Jefferson Medical College in Philadelphia, Pennsylvania, and a masters degree in neuropsychiatry from the University of Michigan. He completed his psychiatry residency at Ypsilanti State Hospital in Michigan and subsequently became an assistant professor of psychiatry at the University of Michigan. Dr. Boyd came to Indiana University School of Medicine in 1939 and took over as head of the Department of Nervous and Mental Diseases. In 1944 he became the first full-time director of the neuropsychiatric unit at Indianapolis City Hospital. At the time he took over the department, there were fifty-five beds with plans to increase the number of beds to about one hundred fifty. In 1948 Dr. Boyd resigned as director of the Department of Neurology and Psychiatry at Indiana University School of Medicine and assumed a position at the Mayo Clinic in Rochester, Minnesota.

# Larue Depew Carter[1-3]

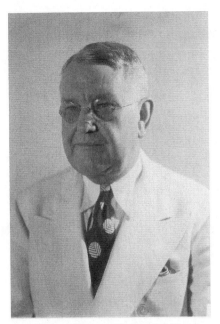

Larue Depew Carter, M.D.

Dr. Carter was born into a Quaker family on March 17, 1880 in Westfield, Indiana. In 1904 he obtained his M.D. degree from the Medical College of Indianapolis. He interned at Indianapolis City Hospital and Philadelphia General Hospital and then took his psychiatry residency at Eastern Indiana Hospital for the Insane in Richmond. He joined the faculty of Indiana University School of Medicine in 1914 and was chief of neuropsychiatry at Indianapolis City Hospital from 1916-19. Dr. Carter was also professor of neurology in the Department of Neuropsychiatry at Indiana University School of Medicine. During his career in Indianapolis, Dr. Carter was on the medical staffs of Methodist, St. Vincent's, Norways, and the Veterans Administration Hospital. He became the director of Norways Hospital after Albert Sterne, M.D., died in 1931 and in 1938 he became the first president of the Indiana Neuropsychiatric Association. He served as chairman of the Indiana Council for Mental Health under Governor Ralph Gates and it was during Carter's tenure that plans were made for the two hundred fifty bed teaching hospital on the west side of Indianapolis that was named after him when it opened in 1952. Dr. Carter died on January 22, 1946 in Indianapolis, Indiana.

An interesting sidelight to Larue Carter is that his portrait hung in the lobby of Carter Hospital on West 10th Street for many years. The artist was Wayman Adams, whose work, along with that of T.C. Steele and other Indiana artists, adorned the walls of the B and C wings of Indianapolis City Hospital. During her lifetime, Carter's wife Ann placed a single red rose on a table beneath the portrait on her husband's birthday. Philip Reed, M.D., adopted son of Larue and Ann Carter, carried on the tradition after Mrs. Carter died.

## Albert Murray DeArmond[1]

Dr. DeArmond was born on January 2, 1899 in Jay County, Indiana. In 1927 he graduated from Indiana University School of Medicine. He interned at Indianapolis City Hospital from 1927-28 and subsequently practiced psychiatry in Indianapolis. He was president of the Indiana Neuropsychiatric Association from 1949-50. He was a staff psychiatrist both at Norways and Methodist Hospitals. Murray had a brilliant mind. After retiring he taught himself how to read Greek. He died on January 2, 1988 in Tucson, Arizona.

## Marian Kendall DeMyer[1-3]

Dr. Marian DeMyer was born in Greensburg, Indiana. Her father, Wilber L. Kendall, was publisher of the *Martinsville Daily Reporter* and a member of the 1972 Indiana Journalism Hall of Fame. Initially Marian worked for her father's newspaper before working during World War II at newspapers in Kansas and Texas. She obtained her undergraduate degree in 1948 and her medical degree in 1952, both from Indiana University.

Marian was married in September 1952 to her now late husband, William DeMyer, M.D., a medical school classmate. Bill and Marian both interned in Michigan, she in Detroit and he at Ann Arbor at the University of Michigan. They returned to Indiana University School of Medicine for their residencies, he in neurology and she in psychiatry.

Bill led a storied career as a child neurologist at Indiana University School of Medicine in Indianapolis. He was named Outstanding Teacher in the Clinical Sciences ten times and received the Golden Apple Teaching Award four times. For many years Bill performed neurology consultations at Larue Carter Memorial Hospital.

Marian's career path led her to Larue D. Carter Memorial Hospital, where she organized a special unit for the study of autistic children. Her research exploded the prevailing belief that infantile autism was caused by a cold, unaffectionate mother and demonstrated that it actually had a neurological basis. Marian published the now classic book, *Parents and Children in Autism.*[1]

## John Thacker Ferguson

A very controversial figure, John Ferguson, M.D., was born on June 4, 1908 in Lafayette, Indiana. Prior to attending medical school Mr. Ferguson held a number of jobs including working in the northern Indiana steel mills, selling insurance, selling whiskey, and being a barman for the Fowler Hotel in Lafayette. As a medical student he had his first heart attack and while recovering became addicted to barbiturates which had been used to quell his anxiety. In 1948 he graduated from Indiana University School of Medicine and began his first postgraduate year as a house officer at Indiana University Medical Center in Indianapolis. During this first year as a house officer he was hospitalized for the first of four eventual hospitalizations for a barbiturate withdrawal psychosis. His last two hospitalizations occurred at the Veterans Administration Hospital and one lasted six months and then other for thirteen. It's unclear whether all of his hospitalizations were related to his barbiturate abuse or some other cause, such as bipolar disorder, since Dr. Ferguson was possessed with boundless energy and maintained very late hours as a busy general practitioner in Hamlet, Indiana.[1]

After his last hospitalization, Dr. Ferguson decided to go into psychiatry and began a psychiatry residency at Logansport State Hospital, where he worked for the next two years. While at Logansport he became heavily involved in trying to improve the conditions for the chronic schizophrenic patients on the back wards. He developed an interest in the emerging trans-orbital lobotomy procedure as practiced by Dr. Walter Freeman (See Chapter 1) and practiced his own lobotomies on the bodies of patients who recently had died. Dr. Ferguson and his colleagues, neurosurgeon John Hetherington, M.D., psychiatrist E. Rogers Smith, M.D., and Logansport State Hospital superintendent John A. Larson, M.D., began studying a series of 232 lobotomy patients which they published in the *Journal of the Indiana State Medical Association*. While in the midst of this series of lobotomies Dr. Ferguson went to a medical meeting in Chicago, met Dr. Freeman, and described what he was doing at Logansport State Hospital. Dr. Freeman reportedly told Dr. Ferguson, "Come back and see me again sonny, when you have done a thousand."[2]

The annual report of 1952-53 for Logansport State Hospital lists Drs. Ferguson, Larson, Smith and Carolyn Pratt, M.D., as members of the Psychosurgery Committee. Dr. Hetherington was listed as a consulting neurosurgeon and Dr. Ferguson as a psychiatric resident. During the 1952-53 year forty-one prefrontal lobotomies and 147 trans-orbital lobotomies were performed.[3] Dr. Hetherington was scheduled to give a paper on psychosurgery at the Central Neuro-Psychiatric Association in October of 1953. The annual report of Logansport State Hospital for the 1953-54 year indicated that a total of 339 lobotomies had been performed, of which 281 were of the trans-orbital type. This number is confusing, however, as later in the report a total of 321 lobotomies were reported as having occurred from March 1952 through June 1954. This same report listed the monthly number of lobotomies performed in addition to the dates of surgery, diagnoses, length of illness, age at surgery, and type of lobotomy for 135 patients who had lobotomies during the 1953-54 year. The report also stated that the neurosurgery program began at Logansport State Hospital in 1949. Reported results showed that twenty percent of the patients had been furloughed or were at the furlough level, sixty-six percent had experienced symptomatic improvement, and fourteen percent had experienced no change in their condition. Eighty-two percent of the patients had been diagnosed with schizophrenia. One death was reported in the series of lobotomies performed in the 1953-54 year.[4] No lobotomies were reported in subsequent annual reports of Logansport State Hospital.

Dr. Ferguson eventually lost favor with the Logansport State Hospital administration. The superintendent pushed for fewer lobotomies and Dr. Ferguson was forced to apologize to the ward staff after he had courageously taken down the grates or partitions that separated patients on a back ward and allowed them to go to the dining room to eat with the other patients. This act of kindness was totally successful but probably could have been handled with much greater tact. Perhaps seeing the writing on the wall and unable to procure any of the emerging psychotropic medications for his patients at Logansport State Hospital, Dr. Ferguson moved on to the Traverse City Hospital in Michigan where he remained the next fourteen years until his death from a heart attack while putting out a minor fire at the hospital.[5]

While at Traverse City Hospital Dr. Ferguson investigated and used many new psychopharmacological agents in the treatment of chronically ill schizophrenics and geriatric patients. These medications included the stimulant methylphenidate, the antihistamine doxylamine, azocyclonol, an anti-hallucinogenic agent, acetylpromazine, a phenothiazine antipsychotic medication, reserpine, an antihypertensive with antipsychotic properties, and 2-ethylcrotonylurea, an antianxiety agent. In just a four-year period Dr. Ferguson was first author on at least sixteen academic articles, some of which wee published in very prestigious journals, such as the *American Journal of Psychiatry, Lancet, Journal of the American Medical Association, Journal of Nervous and Mental Disease,* and the *Annals of the New York Academy of Science.*

## William Paul Fisher[1-3]

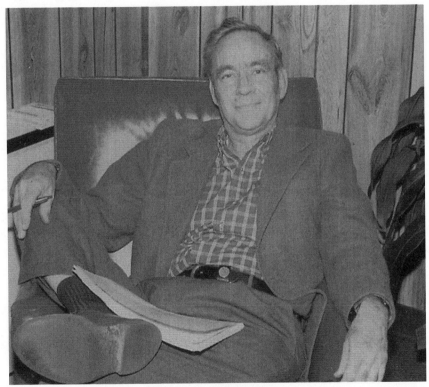

William Paul Fisher, M.D.

Dr. Bill Fisher was born in Massachusetts on October 22, 1929. He graduated from Lebanon Valley College in Annville, Pennsylvania in 1951, earned his M.D. degree from Georgetown University Medical School in 1955, and took his psychiatry training at Brooklyn State Hospital in

New York and Indiana University Hospitals in Indianapolis. Dr. Fisher was a thirty-four-year member of the Department of Psychiatry at Indiana University School of Medicine, where he rose to the rank of professor. An extremely popular psychotherapy supervisor, he received the Psychiatry Residents' Award for Excellence in Teaching four times, more than any other member of the Department of Psychiatry. When Dr. Fisher retired, the Psychiatry Department named its Faculty Excellence in Teaching Award after him.

At least two generations of Indiana University psychiatry residents can recall walking into Dr. Fisher's office for psychotherapy supervision and finding him sitting there with his feet propped up on his desk reading about psychotherapy. He generously loaned out his books on psychotherapy to numerous residents. During the winter he would place corn and other types of birdseed outside his window on top of his air conditioner. Although birds often had first dibs, the numerous squirrels inhabiting the medical center campus were not far behind. Once a squirrel, in search of a noontime meal, landed with such a loud thump on his air conditioner that it scared the daylights out of one of Bill's paranoid patients, who was seated with his back to the window..

Dr. Fisher had a notoriously wry sense of humor. His office was decorated with beautifully carved and painted wooden duck decoys and small stone gargoyles were placed on top of his overflowing book cases. He had a great knack of pointing out his colleagues' foibles by his choice of humorous gifts that he presented at office Christmas parties.

Some of Bill's clinical interests included forensic psychiatry and gender identity disorder. He died of heart failure on February 14, 1998 in St. Luis Obispo, California.

## Ernest J. Fogel[1-3]

Dr. Fogel was born in 1906. He was superintendent of Logansport State Hospital, where he served from 1958-67. While at Logansport Dr. Fogel introduced work therapy programs which resulted in the discharge of a number of long-term patients who had been thought to have been hopelessly incurable. When he left Logansport State Hospital he became chief of the Neuropsychiatry Department at the Veterans Administration Hospital in Murfreesboro, Tennessee. Subsequently he returned to Indiana and became superintendent of Evansville State Hospital until he retired in 1976.

# Richard Noble French[1]

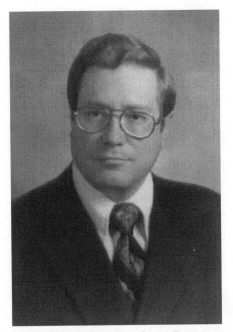

Richard N. French, M.D.

Dr. Dick French was born on February 10, 1932 in Bluffton, Indiana. He obtained his medical degree from Indiana University School of Medicine where he also did his residency training in psychiatry. After serving in the United States Air Force, he returned to the Psychiatry Department at Indiana University School of Medicine where he eventually became full professor. During the first part of his academic career he was director of medical education at Larue Carter Hospital. He left Carter Hospital to become an assistant commissioner in Indiana's Department of Mental Health. When he returned to the university, he served as the medical director of the inpatient adult psychiatry unit at University Hospital. Under his direction, the inpatient unit developed specialty programs, including eating disorders treatment. Leaving that position, he consulted at Midtown Community Mental Health Center for a number of years until his retirement. Dr. French died in October 2005 of complications related to his second heart transplant. He was known for his dedication to teaching and clinical service despite his severe health challenges.

# Herbert Stockton Gaskill[1-2]

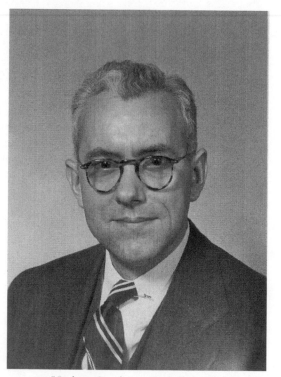

Herbert Stockton Gaskill, M.D.

Dr. Gaskill was born on January 31, 1909. He graduated from Haverford College in 1932 and received his medical degree from the University of Pennsylvania in Philadelphia in 1937. He completed his internship and residency at Philadelphia Hospital. During World War II he spent two years in India as chief of neuropsychiatry. After the war he became assistant professor of psychiatry at the University of Pennsylvania from 1946-49 and began his psychoanalytic training at the Institute of the Philadelphia Psychoanalytic Society. He served as chairman of the Psychiatry Department at Indiana University School of Medicine from 1949-53. While in Indianapolis he continued his psychoanalytic training at the Psychoanalytic Institute of Chicago. After he left Indiana University he went to the University of Colorado to become the Chairman of the Department of Psychiatry. He was also the director of the Colorado Psychoanalytic Institute. Dr. Gaskill died on May 10, 1993 in Denver, Colorado.

# John Howard Greist, Sr.[1]

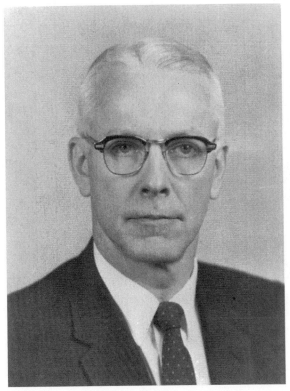

John Howard Greist, M.D.

Dr. Greist was born on February 1, 1906. He was a 1926 graduate of DePauw University and graduated from Indiana University School of Medicine in 1929. He interned at the Indiana University Medical Center from 1929-30. From 1933-35 he took his psychiatry training at Johns Hopkins University in Baltimore, Maryland. Trained as an electroencephalographer at the Mayo Clinic, he established an electroencephalography laboratory at Methodist Hospital in 1947. Dr. Greist was a clinical professor emeritus of psychiatry at Indiana University School of Medicine and was one of Indianapolis' longest practicing private psychiatrists. His colleagues held his psychotherapy skills in high respect. He was an early president of the Indiana Neuropsychiatric Association, forerunner of the Indiana Psychiatric Society. Dr. Greist died on March 5, 1994.

## Hanus Jiri Grosz[1]

Dr. Hanus Grosz was born in Czechoslovakia in 1924. Although his Jewish parents perished in the Nazi Holocaust, he was one of the fortunate children who was exiled at age fifteen to England in the Kindertransport, an effort by allied nations to help save Jewish children. During World War II he served with a Czechoslovakian bomber squadron which was part of the Royal Air Force of England. After the war he returned briefly to Czechoslovakia, but went back to Great Britain to obtain his undergraduate degree at University College in Cardiff and his medical degree at the Welsh National School of Medicine. He immigrated to the United States in the late 1950s.

Dr. Grosz worked nineteen years in the Psychiatry Department at Indiana University School of Medicine and during eight of those years worked at the Roudebush Veterans Administration Hospital. His clinical interests included using hypnosis to treat addictions, teaching hypnosis to psychiatry residents, and utilizing group therapy to help criminal offenders. With his eastern European accent and his Old World manners, he was a colorful and personally powerful figure. After he retired from the university as a professor of psychiatry, Dr. Grosz opened a private practice in Indianapolis and had offices in several other Indiana cities. He died on September 26, 2001.

## Charles Keith Hepburn[1]

Charles Hepburn, M.D., was born on January 31, 1907 in Bloomington, Indiana. He obtained his both his undergraduate and medical from Indiana University. He interned at Indianapolis City Hospital from 1931-32, where he also did a residency in medicine from 1932-34. He obtained his training in psychiatry at Norways Hospital from 1935-36. He practiced both neurology and psychiatry in Indianapolis. Dr. Hepburn was active in teaching psychiatry at Indiana University School of Medicine and was also a president of the Indiana Neuropsychiatric Association. He died on March 12, 1970.

## Frank Frazier Hutchins[1]

Dr. Hutchins was born on February 9, 1870 in Indianapolis, Indiana. He attended Butler University in Indianapolis and Brown University in Providence, Rhode Island. During part of his career he served as chief of the neuropsychiatric service at Walter Reed Hospital in Washington,

D.C. He also had been clinical director of neuropsychiatry for the United States Veterans' Bureau. Dr. Hutchins was professor and chairman of the Department of Nervous and Mental Diseases at Indiana University School of Medicine from 1906-37. He was a prolific writer of scientific articles and studied in Great Britain, France, Germany, and Switzerland. Dr. Hutchins died on September 22, 1942 in Indianapolis.

## Donald H. Jolly[1-2]

Of all the psychiatrists described in this chapter, Dr. Jolly has perhaps the most diverse educational background and clinical/administrative experience. Born in Hamilton, Ontario, Canada, Don obtained his bachelor's degree from McMaster University in Hamilton in 1938. From 1938-42, he undertook graduate studies in electrical engineering at Cornell University in Ithaca, New York. Following his World War II service in the Signal Corps of the Canadian Navy, he pursued and obtained his medical degree from McGill University in Montreal, Quebec, Canada in 1949 under the Canadian equivalent of the United States G.I. bill. He did a rotating internship at Royal Victoria Hospital in Montreal and then completed a pediatric residency at Children's Hospital in Boston, Massachusetts. In 1951 he began work at the Wrentham State School in Massachusetts. He did his psychiatry residency at Boston Psychopathic Hospital. While in Boston, Dr. Jolly worked on epileptic twin studies with William G. Lennox, M.D., a pioneer in the use of electroencephalography in epilepsy. Prior to coming to Indiana in 1957, Dr. Jolly was employed at the Walter E. Fernald State School in Waltham, Massachusetts.

From 1957-67 Dr. Jolly was superintendent at Muscatatuck State Hospital. He recounted these accomplishments while at Muscatatuck: improving the nursing and attendant program with masters level nurses from Indiana University, pre-admission evaluation of waiting list patients and temporary placement of some in respite care to give parents a respite from caretaking during the summer, work with parent's groups such as the Association for Retarded Citizens, the building of the Muscatatuck's chapel and construction of five sixteen-bed treatment cottages for high functioning patients, organization of training rotations for psychiatry residents, medical students, and nurses, improving the speech and hearing program, and hiring more medical and pediatric consultants. During his tenure at Muscatatuck, the hospital obtained grant support for research into obesity in Down's syndrome patients and the screening for abnormal proteins in blood and urine. The hospital was also the site for studies on Crest Toothpaste.

From Muscatatuck, Dr. Jolly went to Pennsylvania where he became their first state commissioner of mental retardation. He then became the acting superintendent at the Pennhurst State School and Hospital in Spring City, Pennsylvania. In 1977 Dr. William Murray, Indiana Commissioner of Mental Health, recruited Dr. Jolly to come to Central State Hospital where he remained until the hospital closed in 1994. While at Central, Don was the Clinical Director for several years and then worked with patients with chronic schizophrenia. When Central State Hospital closed, Dr. Jolly transferred to Carter Hospital where he finally retired in 1997. While at Carter, Don worked with forensic patients who had been sent there for restoration of competency to stand trial.

## Jefferson F. Klepfer[1-2]

Dr. Klepfer was born on April 5, 1905 in Fortville, Indiana. He graduated from Indiana University School of Medicine in 1930 and subsequently took his psychiatry residency at Richmond State Hospital. He then worked at Richmond State Hospital as a staff physician until he went to Central State Hospital in Waupun, Wisconsin in 1936. He eventually became superintendent there until he entered the military service in 1943. He returned from the military to become superintendent of Richmond State Hospital in November 1952, where he remained for the next twenty-three years. Even at the age of seventy, he knew all 1,100 patients at the hospital by name, a truly remarkable feat. Dr. Klepfer died on February 28, 1976 in Richmond.

## Helen P. Langner[1]

Dr. Helen Langner was born on May 9, 1892 in Milford, Connecticut. She graduated from Hunter College in New York City in 1914. As a young college graduate she marched in a women's suffrage rally. After trying an administrative job at St. Luke's Hospital in New York, she decided to attend medical school. During the four years that she attended Yale University Medical School she lived at home in Milford with her parents and daily took the train to New Haven to attend classes. The only woman in her medical school class, she graduated from Yale in 1922. Subsequently she completed a psychiatry residency at Wards Island State Mental Hospital in New York City. She then set up child psychiatry clinics around the country. From 1927-29 she was the first clinical director of a child psychiatry clinic at Indiana University School of Medicine in Indianapolis, but after stock market crashed in 1929, funds dried up for operation of the clinic. In 1931 she assumed the position of medical director of health services at Vassar College. Over the years she was a strong supporter for women in medicine and was named an honorary member of the Class of 1998 at Yale University School of Medicine. She was bestowed this honor because 1998 was the first year that the Yale University entering class in medicine contained more women than men. After spending ten years at Vassar College she opened a private practice in psychiatry in New York City. She eventually retired from private practice and began a second career as a volunteer at the Milford City Health Department. She finally retired at age ninety-eight but continued to live a vibrant life until she died at age 105 on December 10, 1997 at her home in Milford. At her death she was the oldest resident in Milford and was the oldest graduate of Yale University School of Medicine.

### John Augustus Larson[1-5]

Dr. Larson was born in 1892 in Shelbourne, Nova Scotia, Canada. He was a medical student at the University of California. He invented the lie detector in 1921 when consulting with the Berkeley, California Police Department. Dr. Larson trained at the Phipps Clinic at Johns Hopkins University School of Medicine and subsequently became a professor there. He was head of the Arizona State Hospital. From 1949-55 Dr. Larson was superintendent at Logansport State Hospital, during which time he vastly improved the hospital's treatment of the mentally ill by tripling the hospital staff and ending the warehousing of patients. He screened all patients for medical and psychiatric illnesses, brought in surgical and pathology consultants, reactivated the hydrotherapy department, set up a nurses' training center, and established separate wards for the treatment of tuberculosis and alcoholism. He died September 22, 1965 in Nashville, Tennessee.

### Ott Benton McAtee[1]

Dr. McAtee was born in Cadiz, Kentucky on July 23, 1902. He received his undergraduate degree from the University of Kentucky and his medical degree from the Vanderbilt University in Nashville, Tennessee. Prior to coming to Madison State Hospital in 1952 as superintendent, he worked for the Tennessee Valley Authority as director of their mental hygiene program.

He also worked at Overbrook Hospital in Cedar Grove, New Jersey, the New York State Psychiatric Institute, and a Veterans Administration Hospital. Dr. McAtee died on April 18, 1989 in Madison, Indiana.

### Earl William Mericle[1]

Dr. Mericle was born on November 30, 1903 in Anderson, Indiana. He attended Purdue and Butler Universities and graduated from Indiana University School of Medicine in 1934. He interned at Indianapolis City Hospital from 1934-35 and then took his psychiatry residency at Norways Hospital. He completed postgraduate training at the University of Pennsylvania. Dr. Mericle was a president of the Indianapolis Medical Society (1950) and the Indiana State Medical Association (1960). During World War II he was a psychiatrist working under General George Patton in the Fourth Armored Division of the Third Army. According to colleagues he treated many private psychiatric patients at Methodist Hospital and was often at the hospital from early morning until late evening. His daughter, Mary Mericle Ferree, M.D., also became a psychiatrist, specializing in child psychiatry. Dr. Mericle died on March 7, 1979.

### Donald Floyd Moore[1-4]

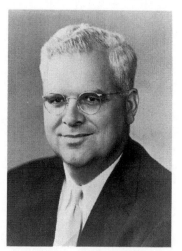

Donald Floyd Moore, M.D.

Dr. Donald Moore was born on July 6, 1914 in Winona, Minnesota. He did his undergraduate training at the University of Michigan in Ann

Arbor, from where he also obtained his M.D. degree in 1938. From 1938-40 he trained in psychiatry at Ypsilanti State Hospital, before serving in the Army during World War II. During the war he saw service in Texas, China, Burma, and Indiana and was discharged as a lieutenant colonel in 1946. After the war he returned to Ypsilanti State Hospital, but in 1948 he became chief of neuropsychiatry at the Veteran's Administration Hospital in Louisville, Kentucky. While in Louisville he was a consultant to the Norton Psychiatric Clinic, Our Lady of the Peace Hospital, Central State Hospital [Kentucky], and the Chrysler Corporation. He also worked as a staff psychiatrist in the Louisville Child Guidance Clinic.

On October 1, 1955 Dr. Moore became superintendent of Larue Carter Memorial Hospital, where he served in this capacity until 1980. He was promoted to professor of psychiatry at Indiana University School of Medicine in 1969. Don published numerous scientific articles on psychiatry, was on the editorial board of *Hospital and Community Psychiatry*, was a long-time examiner for the American Board of Psychiatry and Neurology, and was a founding member of the Association of Medical Superintendents of Mental Hospitals. He consulted at Christian Theological Seminary in Indianapolis and was president of both the Central Neuropsychiatric Association and the Indiana Psychiatric Society.

Keeping with the early tradition of state hospital superintendents who were legally required to live on the hospital grounds, Dr. Moore and his family lived on the fourth floor of Carter Hospital. It must have been very interesting to have been one of the four children of Don and Carolla Moore and to have grown up in a state mental hospital on the edge of metropolitan Indianapolis.

Don was a man of many interests, which included not only many areas of psychiatry, but religion, travel, sailing, fishing, reading, and, of course, gourmet food, an interest which added a number of pounds to his large frame.

Don enjoyed smoking his pipe. His office had many piles of papers and articles, which were kept neatly arranged by his long-time secretary, Doris Chambers. Around the office were many knickknacks, of which the most interesting was the sign, "Time Wounds All Heels." There was, of course, his ever-present coffee pot.

In the center of Don's office was a long conference table and numerous chairs ringed the periphery. On every morning Monday through Friday Don chaired the "morning report." The morning report was supposed to be about the happenings in psychiatry at the Indiana University Medical

Center from 5 PM the previous day until 8 AM the next. However, after hearing from the on-call resident and the night shift nurses, this meeting would often degenerate into a free-for-all discussion about almost any topic imaginable. Sometimes these meetings would continue until 10 AM. A colleague of Don's liked to tell the story about how George Weinland, M.D., chief of one of the adult services, became so bored with the proceedings one morning that he started a small fire in a glass ashtray, which then shattered with a resounding pop!

Don was an accomplished administrator, however. He built Carter Hospital into a fine teaching hospital and the flagship of the Indiana's state public hospitals. He and the Psychiatry Department chairman, John Nurnberger, Sr., were quite adept at obtaining funding, not only for Carter Hospital, but for the entire psychiatry department. For many years Carter Hospital was the primary funding source for salaries of both psychiatry residents and psychology interns.

Dr. Moore died on September 10, 1999.

## Margaret Elaine Morgan

Dr. Morgan was born on June 20, 1913 in Indiana. She received her M.D. degree from the University of Maryland School of Medicine. Her internship was at Grasslands Hospital in Valhalla, New York. Subsequently she trained first as a surgeon at Belleview Hospital in New York City and then further specialized in psychiatry at the New York State Psychiatric Institute. She first set up practice as a private psychiatrist in New York City. In 1950 she returned to Indiana as an assistant professor of psychiatry at Indiana University School of Medicine.[1]

In July 1953, she was appointed Indiana's first commissioner of mental health. Because of the celebrity that this appointment created,[2] she was featured in *Time*,[3] *Look*,[4] *Life*, *Newsweek*, *Vogue*,[5] and the *Police Gazette* magazines in 1955. After her appointment as commissioner, Dr. Morgan, Indiana Governor George North Craig, and Indiana Department of Health director Bertram Groesbeck, Jr., took a tour of Indiana's ten mental health and developmental disabilities facilities. What they found was shocking. At Central State Hospital patients in the men's infirmary were found lying in their excrement. Patients at the Village for Epileptics in New Castle were being fed on seventeen cents a day. At Muscatatuck State School for the Mentally Retarded they found gross malnutrition. Within the next year they added twenty-eight physicians, thirty-one social workers, fifty-one nurses, and five hundred sixty attendants to the state system. When she was appointed as a commissioner, patients were being treated at $1.97 a day and by 1956 this figure had been increased to $3.57 a day. One of her final acts in her position as commissioner was to provide plans for building the Institute for Psychiatric Research on the Indiana University Medical Center campus in Indianapolis.

In her later years Dr. Morgan set up practice as a private psychiatrist in Indianapolis. She died at the age of ninety in Austin, Indiana on January 5, 2004.[6]

## William E. Murray[1]

In 1943 Dr. Murray graduated from Colgate University in Hamilton, New York. In 1949 He obtained his M.D. degree from Syracuse University College of Medicine. He was commissioner of the Indiana Department of Mental Health from 1971-80. During his administration as commissioner he was involved in the establishment of Indiana's system of community mental health centers. Prior to becoming commissioner he had been superintendent of New Castle State Hospital and medical director and assistant superintendent of Madison State Hospital. For eight years he was a surveyor for the Joint Commission on Accreditation of Hospitals. A clinical professor emeritus in psychiatry at Indiana University, Dr. Murray died on July 16, 1998.

## Juul C. Nielsen[1-2]

Dr. Nielsen was the first superintendent of Larue Carter Memorial Hospital. He was born on May 31, 1896 in Langballe, Jutland, Denmark. He immigrated to the United States around 1914. He attended Dana College in Blair, Nebraska and graduated from the University of Nebraska School of Medicine in 1926. He completed his internship at Emanuel Hospital and his psychiatry residency at the University of Colorado Psychiatric Hospital in Denver. In 1938 he was boarded by the American Board of Psychiatry and Neurology.

From 1928-29 Dr. Nielsen engaged in general practice. During the following two years he was a staff physician at Norfolk State Hospital in Nebraska. Then in 1933 he became superintendent of Hastings State Hospital in Ingleside, Nebraska. From 1942-45 Dr. Nielsen served in the United States Army. Following the war, he returned to Hastings State Hospital where he continued as superintendent until 1951 when he was recruited as the first superintendent of Larue Carter Hospital. He remained superintendent at Carter until 1955 when he left to become superintendent of Central State Hospital in Petersburg, Virginia until 1958. He then returned to Hastings and was superintendent there until he retired in 1962. Dr. Nielsen was a member of the Governing Council of the American Psychiatric Association in the early 1950s and was the director of the Indiana Mental Health Council during his sojourn in Indiana. He died on June 2, 1970 in Naples, Florida.

## John Ignatius Nurnberger, Sr.[1-2]

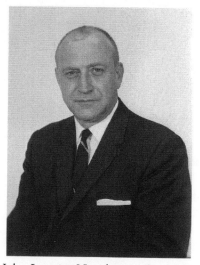

John Ignatius Nurnberger, Sr., M.D.

Dr. John Nurnberger was born in Illinois on April 9, 1916. He graduated from Loyola University in Chicago in 1938 and earned his M.D. degree from Northwestern University Medical School in 1943. He served in World War II and, following the war, held a research fellowship at the Nobel Institute for Cell Research and Genetics in Stockholm, Sweden. Prior to assuming the chair of the Department of Psychiatry at Indiana University School of Medicine in 1956, Dr. Nurnberger was educational and research director at the Institute of Living in Hartford, Connecticut and was on the faculty of Yale University Medical School. John also served as acting dean at Indiana University Medical School from 1964-65. In 1972 he was named distinguished professor of psychiatry at Indiana University School of Medicine. For many years Dr. Nurnberger also served as director of the Institute of Psychiatric Research in

Indianapolis. During his career he was the recipient of many awards and was on several committees at the National Institute of Mental Health. A beloved and skilled teacher, he was unique in championing genetic and biological research in psychiatry while also valuing psychodynamic psychotherapy. One of John's four children, John I. Nurnberger, Jr., M.D., followed in his father's footsteps and became a research psychiatrist in psychiatric genetics and is the current director of the Institute of Psychiatric Research. Dr. John Nurnberger, Sr., died on June 11, 2001.

## Philip Byron Reed, III[1-2]

Dr. Reed was a giant among Indiana psychiatrists. Born April 19, 1906 in Waukon, Iowa, he received his B.Sc. degree from Indiana University in 1928 and his M.D. degree from Indiana University School of Medicine in 1930. He interned at Indianapolis City Hospital from 1930-31. From 1931-32 he was a medicine resident at Indianapolis City Hospital. From 1932-34 he was a psychiatry resident at Indianapolis City Hospital and he completed his psychiatry residency at Norways Hospital from 1934-36.

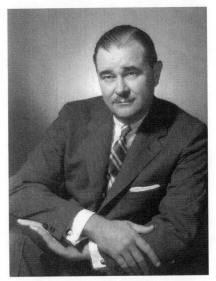

Philip Byron Reed, III, M.D.

Dr. Reed practiced neuropsychiatry for fifty years, thirty-six of them in Indianapolis, where he was assistant superintendent of Indianapolis City Hospital (1932-34) and medical director of Norways Hospital (1946-57). He was chairman of the Neuropsychiatry Department at Methodist

Hospital and was also an associate professor of neuropsychiatry at Indiana University School of Medicine. He was the first medical director of the Marion County Child Guidance Clinic. Dr. Reed held a number of offices in professional organizations including chair of the board of directors of the Indiana Mental Health Association, president of the Indiana Neuropsychiatric Association (1950), vice president of the American Psychiatric Association, and president of the Central Neuropsychiatric Association (1961). After leaving Indianapolis he moved to Florida where he continued to practice psychiatry for another fourteen years. Dr. Reed died in St. Petersburg, Florida on March 13, 1997.

## Nancy Carolynn Arnold Roeske[1-2]

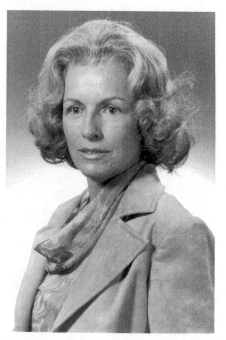

Nancy Carolynn Arnold Roeske, M.D.

The daughter of two physicians, Nancy Roeske was born April 17, 1928 in Minneapolis Minnesota. She graduated from Vassar College, Poughkeepsie, New York in 1950 and obtained her M.D. degree in 1954 from Cornell University Medical College in Ithaca, New York. She began her psychiatry residency in 1955 at Norways Hospital in Indianapolis and finished her residency training at Indiana University School of Medicine in 1964. From

1964-73 she was the director of the Riley Child Guidance Clinic at Riley Hospital in Indianapolis. For many years she was coordinator of medical education in psychiatry for Indiana University School of Medicine. Dr. Roeske and Dr. Clare Assue edited the popular book, *Examination of the Personality*, published in 1969.[3] This book was used for many years to teach Indiana University sophomore medical students how to conduct a mental status examination. Dr. Roeske was president of the Indiana Psychiatric Society from 1981-82. For many years she did child psychiatric consultations for the Indiana School for the Blind. Her research interests involved the role of women in families, especially in women medical students and residents. Dr. Roeske served as a role model for a generation of Indiana women physicians and psychiatrists. She was active on a national level in the American Psychiatric Association and received many awards for her educational and research efforts.

Nancy died in April 1986. The Nancy C.A. Roeske, M.D., Certificate of Recognition for Excellence in Medical Student Education Award, given by the American Psychiatric Association, was established to honor the many years of service that she gave to the American Psychiatric Association.

## Dwight William Schuster

Dr. Dwight Schuster, the "Dean of Indiana psychiatry," was born in 1917 in Shawnee, Ohio. He obtained his bachelor's degree from Butler University in Indianapolis and graduated from Indiana University School of Medicine in 1944. He interned at the Jersey City Medical Center from 1944-45 and continued his training in neuropsychiatry at Methodist Hospital and Norways Hospital in Indianapolis. He was secretary-treasurer of the Indiana Neuropsychiatric Association for many years and was its president from 1963-64. He was also president of the Indianapolis Medical Society from 1967-68 and director of the Psychiatry Department at Methodist Hospital. Dwight is presently emeritus professor of psychiatry at Indiana University School of Medicine. Only recently retired in 2007, his career in psychiatry spanned over sixty years. His knowledge and skill in clinical, administrative, and forensic psychiatry are simply without peer.

## William Leland Sharp[1-3]

Dr. Sharp was born on July 23, 1906 in Greenwood, Indiana. He obtained his M.D. degree from Indiana University School of Medicine in 1930 and interned at Indiana University Hospital. He subsequently completed a three-year residency in psychiatry at Central State Hospital in Indianapolis. Dr. Sharp began a private practice in Anderson, Indiana, but in May 1942 was inducted into the United States Army where he spent the next three and a half years. During his first eighteen months of service he was stationed at Darnall General Hospital in Danville, Kentucky where he treated psychiatric casualties from various World War II fronts. Subsequently he was assigned to the 99th Infantry Division and trained for ten months at Camp Maxey in Texas. Following his training, he served under General Hodges in the battles of the Ardennes, Remagan bridgehead, and the Rhur pocket in Belgium and Germany. During this time he treated psychiatric casualties in a mobile division hospital near the front lines. Following V-E Day, he served four months under General Patton's 3rd Army. In January 1946 Dr. Sharp resumed his private practice in Anderson, Indiana. It wasn't until the mid-1960s that other psychiatrists began to join Dr. Sharp in Anderson. Although he closed his office in 1983, at the ripe old age of eighty Dr. Sharp was still engaged in part-time consulting three days a week. He died in September 1994.

### Patricia Haig Sharpley[1]

Dr. Pat Sharpley was born on January 11, 1932 in Peterborough, England. In 1955 she graduated from the Royal Free Hospital School of Medicine. She interned at Memorial Hospital in Watford, England from 1955-56 and then took her psychiatry residency at Louisville General Hospital, Vanderbilt University, and the University of Minnesota Hospital from 1957-61. In 1969 she became chief of the female service at Larue Carter Memorial Hospital and when the male and female services were combined she became chief of the adult service where she remained until shortly before she died on May 16, 1997. Pat will ever be remembered for her English accent, efficiently proper administrative abilities, and funny stories about the differences between English and American slang. A member of the Department of Psychiatry at Indiana University School of Medicine, she attained the rank of associate professor. She was quite active in professional organizations including the American Psychiatric Association, Indiana Psychiatric Society, and the Central Neuropsychiatric Association.

### James E. Simmons[1-2]

Dr. Jim Simmons was born on July 13, 1923 in Toledo, Ohio. He was a 1945 graduate of the University of Toledo and in 1947 obtained his M.D.

degree from Ohio State University. He interned at St. Vincent's Hospital in Toledo, Ohio in 1948 and from 1951-53 was a psychiatry resident at the Menninger Foundation in Topeka, Kansas. From 1953-57 Jim was the director of the Marion County Child Guidance Clinic in Indianapolis.

Dr. Simmons was a thirty-four-year member of the Psychiatry Department at Indiana University School of Medicine and was named Arthur Richter Professor of Child Psychiatry in 1979. His book, *Psychiatric Examination of Children,*[3] became the handbook of how to perform a psychiatric child examination. This book went through four editions and was printed in five different languages.

As child psychiatrist, Suzanne Blix, M.D., so aptly said in her memorial resolution to Dr. Simmons, he dearly loved children, not only his own eight children, but all children, especially the ones that he treated with so much compassion. She said,

> "A lasting picture of Jim will always be that of him sitting in his office, interviewing a young child, with family present and almost always being able to get at the core of the problem. He could read a child like a book and then be able to use his demonstrative techniques in order to teach others how to pursue interview technique in the same manner."[2]

From 1975-88 Jim was the Director of Child Psychiatry in the Psychiatry Department at Indiana University School of Medicine. He was a tireless advocate for the humane treatment of children both on local and national levels. Jim died on August 30, 1998.

## Joyce Graham and Iver Francis Small

No list of prominent Indiana psychiatrists would be complete without this dynamic duo. Joyce was born in Edmonton, Alberta, Canada. She graduated summa cum laude from the University of Saskatchewan in 1951 and obtained her M.D. degree from the University of Manitoba in 1956. She did a rotating internship at Winnipeg General Hospital in 1956 and her psychiatry residency at Ypsilanti State Hospital in Michigan from 1956-59. She completed her M.S. in neurology at the University of Michigan. Prior to coming to Larue Carter Memorial Hospital as clinical director of laboratories in 1965, Joyce worked at the Ypsilanti State Hospital, University of Oregon Medical School, and the Malcolm

Bliss Mental Health Center and City Hospital in St. Louis. She was on the faculties of the University of Michigan, University of Oregon Medical School, and Washington University School of Medicine.

Iver was born in Saskatchewan, Canada, obtained his B.A. from the University of Saskatchewan in 1951, M.D. from the University of Manitoba in 1954, and M.S. in psychiatry from the University of Michigan in 1960. From 1953-54 he did his internship at St. Boniface General Hospital in Manitoba, Canada. From 1954-58 he did his psychiatry residency at Selkirk Hospital for Mental Disease in Selkirk, Canada and Ypsilanti State Hospital in Michigan. Joyce and Iver met at the University of Saskatchewan and were married in 1954. Iver was on the faculties of both the University of Oregon Medical School and Washington University School of Medicine. Both Joyce and Iver are boarded in General Psychiatry. Joyce is a certified electroencephalographer and Iver is a certified hospital administrator.

During their training Joyce and Iver had the choice of either obtaining an M.S. degree or personal psychoanalysis. In retrospect for their storied careers, they wisely chose to obtain their M.S. degrees while in Michigan. While at Washington University in St. Louis they met Lucy King, M.D., who also came to the Indiana University School of Medicine faculty years later.

After coming to Carter Hospital in 1965 Joyce and Iver's careers diverged. Joyce took over as director of clinical laboratories and ran the clinical laboratory and electroencephalography laboratory. After several years doing research she took over ward B2, which had been a teaching "museum" ward and turned it into an outstanding research service. Iver became Assistant Superintendent Medical and took over the supervision of electroconvulsive therapy. Over their many years at Carter they collaborated on many research projects including studies of electroconvulsive therapy and clinical trials of lithium carbonate, clozapine, and numerous other psychiatric medications. Both have won many awards which are too numerous to mention. Both of the Drs. Small are now retired.

### Edwin Rogers Smith[1]

Dr. Smith was born April 5, 1892 in Richmond, Indiana. He was the son of Samuel E. Smith, M.D., superintendent of Richmond State Hospital, where E. Rogers Smith grew up. He graduated from Indiana University in 1914 and received his M.D. degree from the University of Michigan in 1918. Dr. Smith interned at the University of Michigan and then did his psychiatry residency at Boston Psychopathic Hospital and the Phipps Psychiatric Clinic at John Hopkins Hospital in Baltimore. He began practice at the Phipps Clinic and then moved to Indianapolis in 1922 where he practiced psychiatry for the next fifty years. He was on the staff at Norways Hospital and was president of the Indiana Neuropsychiatric Association in 1940. He was a professor at Indiana University School of Medicine. From 1938-51 he was chief of the medical staff at the Indianapolis Motor Speedway. Dr. Smith died on July 2, 1972 in Indianapolis. He was known was a colorful man who bragged about being born in a state mental hospital.

## William C. Strang[1]

William Strang was born on November 26, 1912 in Indiana. Both his undergraduate and medical degrees were from Indiana University. He was assistant medical director at Larue Carter Hospital from 1957-63. After leaving Carter Hospital he was in private practice in Indianapolis for many years. For five years he was head of the Psychiatry Department at Methodist Hospital. Dr. Strang died on October 4, 2002.

## Wallace Raymond Van Den Bosch[1]

Dr. Van Den Bosch was born on June 28, 1920 in Bradenton, Florida. He obtained both his undergraduate and medical degrees from Indiana University. From 1952-56 he was superintendent of Norman Beatty Hospital in Westville, Indiana but resigned this position because he disagreed with Governor George Craig's decision to have the Indiana State Prison warden take over administration of the maximum security building for insane criminals.[2] Following his resignation as superintendent, Wally Van Den Bosch opened a private practice in psychiatry in Lafayette, Indiana where he practiced until 1982. A little known fact about him is that he and his wife owned several Tennessee Walking Horses. He subsequently worked at the Caylor Nickel Clinic in Bluffton Indiana until he retired in 1991. Dr. Van Den Bosch died on January 30, 2006.

## Walter Crowe VanNuys[1-2]

The son of a physician, Dr. Van Nuys was born on April 1, 1877 in Montgomery County, Indiana. After attending Hanover College for a year, he graduated from Kansas University. He attended Rush Medical School at the University of Chicago and then was employed at the

Kansas State Hospital in Topeka, Kansas for four years. He subsequently was superintendent of the Kansas School for the Feeble Minded prior to returning to Indiana in order to superintend the Indiana Village for Epileptics in New Castle in 1906. Dr. VanNuys was superintendent there until he retired in April 1952. He died in December 1955 in Dayton, Ohio at the home of his son. One of Dr. Nuys' sons, John D. VanNuys, M.D., became dean of Indiana University Medical School in Indianapolis where the medical school building now bears his name.

## George C. Weinland[1]

Dr. George Weinland was born on January 20, 1923 in Hope, Indiana. He received both his undergraduate degrees and medical degrees from Indiana University. He subsequently completed a psychiatry residency at Indiana University School of Medicine in Indianapolis. After his residency he worked at Carter Hospital for several years as assistant superintendent. In 1960 he moved back to Bartholomew County, Indiana and became the first psychiatrist in Columbus, Indiana. He was the first director of the Bartholomew County Mental Health and Child Guidance Clinic, which later became Quinco Community Mental Health Center. Dr. Weinland died on September 9, 2004 in Columbus, Indiana.

## Clifford Leland Williams[1-4]

Dr. Williams was born in 1901 in Muncie, Indiana. He received his undergraduate degree from Indiana University and in 1926 he received his medical degree from Indiana University School of Medicine. He took post graduate training in psychiatry for two years at Philadelphia General Hospital. In 1946 he became the first director of the Indiana Mental Health Council, the forerunner of the state's Department of Mental Health. Dr. Williams was superintendent of Central State Hospital from 1952-66. Prior to coming to that position he also had been a superintendent of Logansport State Hospital. Dr. Williams died on October 1, 1967 in Indianapolis.

## James J. Wright[1-2]

Dr. James Wright was born on June 25, 1935 in Fowler, Indiana. He graduated from St. Joseph's College in Rensselaer, Indiana in 1955 and from the Stritch School of Medicine at Loyola University in Chicago in

1959. After his internship at Cincinnati General Hospital, he completed a psychiatry residency at Indiana University School of Medicine in 1968. He joined the staff of Marion County General Hospital and then became medical director of Midtown Community Mental Health Center when it opened in 1969. During Dr. Wright's twenty-two-year tenure as medical director at Midtown, the center added partial hospitalization, satellite neighborhood clinics, addiction services, and a crisis intervention service. After he stepped down as medical director, Jim continued to work at Midtown until he retired in 2000. Dr. Wright is best known as a compassionate physician and an ever-so-calm administrator. He had a subtle sense of humor. Besides being a psychiatrist Jim was an accomplished pianist and wildflower gardener. He died on April 17, 2001.

CHAPTER 14

# Notable Non Psychiatrists from Indiana

"There were epileptics, raving maniacs, cleptomaniacs and
melancholia. There were those tending to suicide, religious
fanatics, sex crazy, and dangerous ones who were cruel
and cunning."

Carrie E. Lively.
Reminiscences of a state mental hospital attendant.
*Indiana Medical History Quarterly*, 11,
March 1983, p. 13.

The history of Indiana psychiatry would not be complete without
mentioning non-psychiatrists since psychiatry is a collaborative profession
working with other health professionals including psychologists, social
workers, neurologists, neurosurgeons, chaplains, nurses, neuroscientists,
and other allied health professionals such as occupational, recreational,
vocational, art, and music therapists. Sometimes it truly takes a village to
help someone who is emotionally ill. This chapter's short list mentions only
a few of these notable individuals.

## Morris Herman Aprison[1]

Morrie was born in Milwaukee, Wisconsin in 1923. He received his
bachelor's degree in chemistry, master's degree in physics, and Ph.D.
degree in biochemistry, all at the University of Wisconsin. From 1952-
56 he was chief of biophysics at Galesburg State Hospital in Galesburg,
Illinois. He came to the Institute of Psychiatric Research in Indianapolis
in 1956. During his years at the Institute he taught a graduate course in
neurochemistry and maintained an extremely active research program
studying neurotransmitters. His work regarding glycine and gamma-
aminobutyric acid is known and admired throughout the world. From

1974-78 he was director of the Institute. Although he retired in 1993, he continued his research until July 2000. He published a prodigious number of papers. In order to honor him, in 2006 the Morris H. Aprison Lectureship in Biological Psychiatry was established by the Department of Psychiatry at Indiana University School of Medicine. Morrie died on December 2, 2007 in Indianapolis.

## Malcolm B. Ballinger[1-2]

Rev. Ballinger was born on December 30, 1912 in Henry County, Indiana. A gifted musician, he played the trumpet with the Chautauqua the summer following his graduation from high school. In 1934 he graduated from Indiana University in Bloomington, Indiana. He then obtained both the A.M. and S.T.B. degrees from the Boston University School of Theology. His A.M. thesis was entitled, "The use of religion by certain abnormal personalities in escaping problems of life." Malcolm was one of the early pioneers of the idea that certain forms of religious expression were more mature than others. In 1938 he was ordained as an elder in the Methodist Episcopal Church. He served as a minister in Hermiston, Oregon and in 1943 joined the United States Army as a chaplain. During his service in the Army, Chaplain Ballinger served in England, Alaska, California, and the Philippines. Following WWII he obtained advanced training in hospital chaplaincy at Boston University. While there he adopted Carl Roger's client-centered approach to psychotherapy. While avoiding the usual social interaction among seminary students, Malcolm managed to read the entire works of Sigmund Freud. In 1947 he was named director of clinical pastoral training at the University of Michigan Medical Center. After twenty years in Michigan and training over 500 seminary students in pastoral counseling, he assumed a similar position at the Buchanan Counseling Center at Methodist Hospital in Indianapolis, Indiana in 1968. From there he went to Larue Carter Memorial Hospital in Indianapolis as the full time chaplain from 1973-77. While at Buchanan he wrote the *Pastoral Counseling Guidebook* for the center. Following his "retirement" from Carter Hospital he worked at the Buchanan Counseling Center again and became director of the counseling center at the Chapel Hill United Methodist Church in Indianapolis.

## Norman Madrid Beatty[1-3]

Norman Beatty was born in Indianapolis, Indiana on March 30, 1902. He obtained his undergraduate degree from Indiana University in 1925 and his

M.D. degree in 1927. He interned at Indianapolis City Hospital and then began the private practice of dermatology. Eventually he became associate professor of dermatology at Indiana University School of Medicine. He was chairman of the Indianapolis Chamber of Commerce Health Committee and helped institute the milk ordinance. During WWII he took an interest in treating venereal diseases and eventually became the director of the Indianapolis Public Health Center where venereal diseases were treated. He helped eliminate prostitution from Indianapolis. He was partly responsible for the formation of the Indiana Council for Mental Health, the forerunner of the Department of Mental Health. He became council president and was instrumental in the building of Larue Carter Memorial Hospital as well as improving mental health care at the Indiana State Prison and the Marion County Jail. Dr Beatty died on December 6, 1948 in Indianapolis. He was recognized posthumously for his work in psychiatry when in 1952 the Northern Indiana Hospital for the Insane was named after him.

### Joyce Bowman

Joyce's career as a psychiatric nurse spanned forty-five years. Her psychiatric career began as a student at Norways Hospital, then as a newly graduated R.N. at Richmond State Hospital, and finally at Carter Hospital where she retired in 1998.

Joyce recalled as a nursing student at Indiana University in Indianapolis that her psychiatric rotation at Norways Hospital lasted twelve weeks. At the time most nursing students lived in the Ball Residence Hall on the medical center campus. During their psychiatric rotations at Norways they were chauffeured by cab between the two facilities. While at Norways Joyce witnessed insulin coma therapy and electroconvulsive therapy, which at the time was given without benefit of anesthesia or muscle relaxants. At least one of her classmates witnessed hydrotherapy while at Norways. Another of her classmates recalled a patient there who wiped off all of his pills with toilet paper each morning before he would swallow them. Since Norways was a private hospital, the food was very good but only one dessert was allowed per person!

Ms Bowman graduated from nursing school in 1954 and immediately started work at Easthaven or Richmond State Hospital where she was assigned as the only R.N. to the afternoon shift. At the time, there were only seven registered nurses for a hospital population of fourteen hundred patients. These nurses were only assigned to the medical hospital and receiving wards, leaving the "back wards" staffed only by attendants who "ran the show." At the time the patient food was not very good, according to Joyce. Patients often only had bread and gravy for breakfast and once she received only twenty-six hot dogs to feed supper to thirty patients.

Joyce left Easthaven to get married, moved to Texas, and became a surgical nurse. She returned to psychiatric nursing when she joined Carter Hospital in 1988. As a ward nurse she worked on both adult wards B1 and E2. Her re-entry into psychiatric nursing after thirty-three years must have been somewhat like Sleeping Beauty waking up after a hundred-year slumber, because the changes in psychiatric treatment over those years were vast. When Joyce left psychiatric nursing at Richmond State Hospital, Milltown, a minor tranquilizer, had just been introduced and the world's first major tranquilizer, Thorazine, had not yet been introduced to Easthaven. When she returned to psychiatric nursing at Carter Hospital in 1988, there were numerous antipsychotic, anxiolytic, and antidepressant medications from which to choose. Electroconvulsive therapy was being given in a much more humane manner and insulin coma therapy and hydrotherapy had gone the way of the dinosaur. "The patients were the same," said Joyce, and she very much enjoyed working with them and seeing them get well.

## Walter L Bruetsch[1-3]

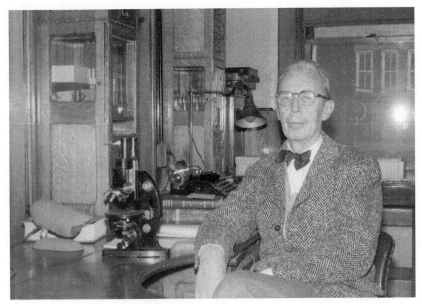

Walter L. Bruetsch, M.D.

Dr. Bruetsch was born on November 25, 1896 in Heidelberg, Germany. In 1922 he received his M.D. degree in Freiberg, Germany. Upon persuasion of Dr. Max Bahr, he came to Indianapolis in 1924 and worked as a research pathologist at Central State Hospital. From 1924-67 he was a member of the Department of Neurology at Indiana University School of Medicine where he was ultimately promoted to full professor. Dr. Bruetsch introduced the use of malarial treatment, first discovered by Dr. Wagner-Jauregg, to individuals suffering from cerebral syphilis. Dr. Bruetsch also introduced the use of electroconvulsive therapy for schizophrenia at Central State Hospital. After retiring, Dr. Bruetsch moved to Santa Barbara, California where he died on January 31, 1977.

## Catherine Eversole

Ms Eversole's career spanned the closing of one state hospital, the move to community care for chronic patients, and the downsizing and upgrading of another state hospital. She has seen it all. A graduate with a bachelor's degree in social work at Eastern Carolina University, Ms Eversole began work in October 1977 at Logansport State Hospital. Although she continued to work at Logansport until June 1988, she spent much of her time living in Warsaw, Indiana and working at the Bowen Community Mental Health Center while handling a family care program in private and group homes. When Norman Beatty hospital closed in the late 1970s, the psychiatric patients housed there moved to other state hospitals and Ms Eversole was witness to the many large vans that carried Norman Beatty's patients to other hospitals.

Eventually Ms Eversole obtained her master's degree in social work from Indiana University Purdue University in Indianapolis (IUPUI). While taking a weekend program in social work at IUPUI for two years, she lived at Logansport State Hospital in an apartment, all for $29 a month.

In 1988 Ms Eversole began work at Evansville State Hospital. She recalls the "old building," completed in 1945, which had medical/geriatric patients on the second floor, women patients on the third floor, men patients on the fourth floor, and substance abuse patients on the fifth floor. In 2003 she and the rest of the staff and patients moved into the present building where she is currently a senior social work supervisor.

## Ezra Vernon Hahn[1-2]

Dr. Hahn was born on October 23, 1891 in the Brightwood neighborhood of Indianapolis, Indiana. He graduated from Wabash College in Crawfordsville, Indiana in 1913. After graduation he taught high school chemistry at Shortridge High School in Indianapolis. In 1920 he graduated from Indiana University School of Medicine in Bloomington, Indiana. From 1922-27 he trained in general and neurosurgery at Robert Long Hospital in Indianapolis. Although he was a surgeon, Dr. Hahn had an immense interest in neuropsychiatry and commuted to the Chicago Psychoanalytic Institute for his personal psychoanalysis. In 1939 and again from 1947-49 he was president of the Indiana Neuropsychiatric Association. Some meetings were held at his home and farm on Eagle Creek near Indianapolis. Besides discussing business, activities included hiking, fishing, playing horseshoes, wood chopping, and milking cows. Dr. Hahn died on October 16, 1959 in Indianapolis.

## Alfred Charles Kinsey[1-3]

Alfred Kinsey, a professor of entomology at Indiana University in Bloomington, Indiana was an unlikely candidate to become one of the greatest sex researchers in the United States. He was born on June 23, 1894 in Hoboken, New Jersey. His father was a professor at the Stevens Institute of Technology and was a devout member of the local Methodist church. While in high school Kinsey developed an interest in biology, but, bowing to the demands of his father, he attended the Stevens Institute of Technology for his first two years of college and then transferred to Bowdoin College in Maine. In 1916 Kinsey was inducted into Phi Beta Kappa and graduated magna cum laude with degrees in biology and psychology. He received his Sc.D. degree in 1919 from Harvard University. Kinsey's doctoral dissertation was on the gall wasp. In fact, he, his students, colleagues, and even some family members obsessively collected 3,500,000 specimens of this insect over twenty-five years and added to Harvard's already burgeoning collection of eighteen million insects. He was especially interested in the mating practices of the gall wasp and this interest probably prepared him to study human sexology.

Kinsey joined the faculty of Indiana University as an assistant professor of Zoology in 1920. During his early years at the university he wrote a number of biology texts. In 1938 he began teaching a marriage course and his research interests eventually led him to begin collecting data on human sexual behavior. He and his colleagues did over eighteen thousand interviews of individuals regarding their sexual practices. He developed the Kinsey Scale, a scale measuring sexual orientation. Kinsey and his colleagues eventually published "*Sexual Behavior in the Human Male*" in 1948[4] and "*Sexual Behavior in the Human Female*" in 1953.[5]

In 1947 Kinsey and colleagues founded the Institute for Research in Sex, Gender and Reproduction at Indiana University. This institute, which continues to this day, is now known as the Kinsey Institute for Research in Sex, Gender, and Reproduction. Julia Heiman, Ph.D., is the current director.

As might be imagined, living and working on sexuality in the middle of America's Bible belt, Kinsey provoked a storm of controversy, which continues to this day. Some of the research techniques used by Kinsey and colleagues have been subjected to intense scrutiny. While working at Indiana University, Kinsey's academic freedom to do research and publish was protected by then president Herman Wells. Kinsey died on August 25, 1956.

## Eugene E. Levitt[1]

Eugene ("Gene") Levitt was a colorful personality. He was born on November 5, 1921 in New York City. In 1948 he received his undergraduate degree from City University in New York. He obtained his master's degree from Columbia University in 1950 and then his Ph.D. in psychology from Columbia in 1952.

In 1952 Dr. Levitt began his academic career as a research assistant professor at the University of Iowa. He was director of research at the Illinois Institute of Juvenile Research from 1955-57. Subsequently he came to the Psychiatry Department at Indiana University School of Medicine where he was director of the Section on Psychology from 1957-87. He attained the rank of full professor and even after his retirement in 1991 he remained active, especially in scheduling speakers for Psychiatry Grand Rounds.

Dr. Levitt was extremely productive academically. In 1957 he established one of the first psychology internship programs approved by the American Psychological Association. He wrote over two hundred scientific articles, book chapters, and books. His academic interests were quite varied and included hypnosis, sexual response and dysfunction, and personality assessment using the Minnesota Multiphasic Personality Inventory and the

Rorschach. Over his career he received numerous awards from a variety of organizations.

## Carrie Lively[1]

Carrie Lively (1871-1957) began work at the Central Indiana Hospital for the Insane in about 1899 while Dr. George Edenharter was superintendent. While there she worked on ward twenty-one which contained severely ill psychiatric patients. She worked with Sarah Stockton, M.D. She witnessed the cruelty of some attendants, one of whom slapped a patient and probably smothered her to death with a wet towel. She saw another patient beat an elderly patient. She enjoyed the beautiful hospital grounds on her evenings off. Unfortunately she was fired by Dr. Edenharter for a minor infraction of the evening pass rules.

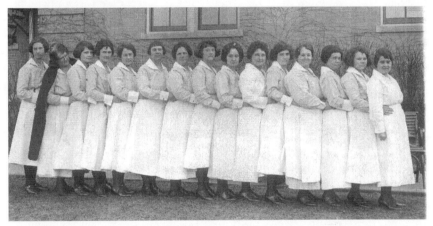

Psychiatric Attendants, Madison State Hospital, Madison, Indiana

After being fired, Miss Lively returned home and eventually secured a job as a maid in Indianapolis. Wanting to return to a hospital attendant job, she applied at the state hospitals in Evansville, Logansport, and Richmond. She was hired at Easthaven in Richmond and very much enjoyed working under Samuel Smith, M.D., the hospital's superintendent. While at Easthaven she witnessed no cruelty towards patients. It seemed to her that Dr. Smith took a much more active role in looking after the welfare of the hospital patients than had Dr. Endenharter at the Central Indiana Hospital for the Insane. She resigned her job in June 1902 to marry an old sweetheart who had recently become widowed.

## Marcia Lurie

Ms Lurie received her AB degree in sociology from Butler University in 1959 and her BS degree in occupational therapy from the Indiana University School of Allied Health Sciences in Indianapolis in 1962. She eventually completed a MS degree in counseling at Butler University/ Christian Theological Seminary in the late 1970s.

Her several degrees prepared her well for her chosen profession of psychiatric occupational therapy. Her first contact with psychiatry was through a three-month rotation in the occupational therapy department at Larue Carter Memorial Hospital in Indianapolis around 1960. After her graduation from the School of Allied Health Sciences she was hired as an occupational therapist at Marion County General Hospital in Indianapolis where she worked from 1962-78 with patients who were too medically ill to be placed on the psychiatry unit. These patients were often hospitalized for lengthy periods on the obstetrics, orthopedics, and coronary care units.

Following her work at General Hospital, Marcia was employed for six months at Central State Hospital in Indianapolis. While at Central she worked in the Evans Building with patients who had mental retardation and developmental disabilities. Most of her work involved teaching patients how to complete their activities of daily living, such as bathing and eating. Of particular note was a feeding program for patients known for choking from bolting their food.

In 1980 Ms Lurie began work in the occupational therapy department at Methodist Hospital in Indianapolis. She became head of the department in 1985, but around 1992-93 the occupational therapy and recreational therapy departments were combined into a new activities therapy department. Marcia continued to direct that department until she retired in 2001. During her years at Methodist Hospital, Marcia watched the length of stay on the psychiatry unit drop from four to six weeks to about five days. When she first arrived the emphasis was on various crafts, such as ceramics and leatherworking, and by the time she left, the emphasis was on various forms of group therapy, such as anger management.

## Victor Milstein[1]

Vic was born in Brooklyn, New York in the late 1920s. He graduated from Brooklyn College in 1951 and received his master's degree from New York City College in 1952. He completed his Ph.D. in psychology from the University of Oregon in 1959 and did his psychology internship at the University of Iowa. In 1965 he completed an advanced course in encephalography in Austria. Over the succeeding years he authored numerous papers, often in conjunction with Drs. Joyce and Iver Small at Carter Hospital. His primary areas of research were electroencephalography and electroconvulsive therapy. Vic died on April 5, 2009 in Indianapolis.

## Ruth Rogers[1-2]

Ruth Rogers, Social Worker of the Year in Central Indiana in 1972, was born near Chatfield, Ohio. She obtained her undergraduate degree from Taylor University in Upland, Indiana and in 1952 obtained her master's degree in social work from the Indiana University Division of Social Service. Subsequently she trained at the Cincinnati Family Institute. Prior to going to Larue Carter Memorial Hospital in 1958 she worked in the Indianapolis Children's Guardian Home and Indianapolis Public Schools. After arriving at Carter Hospital, Ruth worked on the Women's Service for two years and then the Adolescent Service for two years. She eventually became assistant director of the Social Work Department and in 1962 was named director. After she "retired" from Carter in 1990, she became director of the Suburban East Pastoral Counseling Center in Indianapolis. Ruth has taught social work at Marion College in Indianapolis and the IUPUI School of Social Work.

## Norman Skole[1]

One of the most notable leaders of the Indiana Mental Health Association was Norman Skole, who was Executive Director of the Marion County Mental Health Association for thirty-three years. After World War II Mr. Skole obtained his undergraduate degree in social work at Purdue University and completed his master's degree in social work at Indiana University. He then worked for several years as a social worker at Larue Carter Memorial Hospital. From 1959-92 he was Executive Director of the Marion County Mental Health Association. It was under his leadership that the well-known Christmas Gift Lift was created to give Christmas presents to the hospitalized mentally ill people. Mr. Skole was also instrumental in establishing halfway houses for people who had been discharged from state hospitals. He helped establish a suicide prevention hotline in Indianapolis, the first in the United States. Mr. Skole also served as president of the national Mental Health Association.

## Samuel Edwin Smith[1-3]

Dr. Smith was born on August 31, 1861 in Gosport, Indiana. He graduated from Indiana University in 1882 and obtained his M.D. degree from the University of Louisville in 1884. For the next four years he practiced general medicine in Gosport. From 1888-91 he was a staff physician at the Northern Indiana Hospital for the Insane in Logansport. From 1891 to 1923 he was medical superintendent at the Indiana Hospital for the Insane in Richmond. While Dr. Smith was at Richmond State Hospital, the hospital grew from 392 patients and seventeen buildings on 208 acres of land to 951 patients and forty-four buildings on 983 acres. The surrounding farm fields were transformed to a beautiful campus by the planting of numerous trees and shrubs.

In 1910 Dr. Smith was president of the Indiana Board of Charities and Correction and from 1914-15 was president of the American Medico-Psychological Association, forerunner of the American Psychiatric Association. Dr. Smith was helpful in selecting sites for other Indiana institutions including Madison State Hospital, the Indiana State Farm in Putnamville, and New Castle State Hospital. In 1923 Dr. Smith was appointed provost for Indiana University School of Medicine in Indianapolis. Along with other influential citizens, Dr. Smith was responsible for the building of Riley Hospital for Children on the Indiana University Medical Center campus. In 1919 he drafted the voluntary admission law for Indiana state mental hospitals. He was the originator of the farm colony concept for the treatment of mental illness and mental disabilities. Dr. Smith died of heart disease in May 1928 at his home in Indianapolis.

## Arthur Sterne

Art was born in Hudson Falls, New York. Shortly after his birth, his family moved south to Savannah, Georgia for several years and then further south to Jacksonville, Florida where he grew to adulthood. He obtained his bachelor's and master's degrees at the University of Florida in Gainesville. Subsequently he began his trek back north and obtained his Ph.D. in 1961 at Vanderbilt University in Nashville, Tennessee. He moved further north to Larue Carter Hospital in Indianapolis where he did his psychology internship under the tutelage of Herb Nichols, Ph.D. and George Siskind, Ph.D.

After his internship at Carter Hospital, Art joined the staff and continued there until he retired in 1996. He became chief of the

Psychology Department in 1967. Art started Indiana's first American Psychological Association approved internship at Carter Hospital. This internship was later combined with the psychology internship at Indiana University School of Medicine. During the mid to late 1970s Dr. Sterne and colleagues conducted and published a follow-up study of patients who were hospitalized at Carter Hospital. Despite being born a Yankee and living in Indiana nearly fifty years, Art still has a slightly southern accent.

## CHAPTER 15

# Laws

Prosecutor: "Well, Dr. Smith, with credentials such as you have I wonder if you could give the jury your opinion as to whether you are sane or insane?"

Dr. Smith: "Hell, I have an opinion in general I am about as insane as you are. In cases such as this it helps."

Paul H. Buchanan, Jr.
Courting disaster: Recollections of an Indiana judge about Dr. E. Rogers Smith.
*Indiana Medicine*, 78(8), 1985, p. 660.

### Selected Mental Health Laws of Indiana

Over the years The Indiana General Assembly has passed a number of laws dealing with mental health issues. These laws have included laws establishing the state mental hospital system, the commitment of patients to these hospitals, and the building of a hospital for the criminally insane. This chapter discusses some of the more important laws.

"An Act Concerning Insane Persons." This 1815 law of the Indiana Territory was the first law regarding the "insane" in Indiana. The law provided that if a person was suspected of being insane that the court should direct the sheriff of the county to summon "twelve of the most intelligent men in the county, one of whom at least shall be a physician" to choose a time and meeting place to "inspect such insane person." After their inspection and the testimony of the parties involved they were to decide whether the person was insane and whether he or she could care for their property. If the person was insane, the court was to appoint three persons to act as guardians of the person and estate.[1] A similar law was enacted by the 1818 Indiana Legislature in Corydon, Indiana.[2] This 1818 law was amended in 1840.[3]

"An act to provide for the procuring of a suitable site for the erection of a State Lunatic Asylum." In 1845 the Indiana General Assembly realized that the state should provide a suitable site for a public psychiatric facility. Prior to the opening of the Indiana Hospital for the Insane in 1848, persons who were insane were kept at home or housed in county poor houses or jails. This 1845 act appointed John Evans, Livingston Dunlap, and James Blake as the board of commissioners charged with selecting a suitable site, "not exceeding two hundred acres," for a "state lunatic asylum." The land was not to cost more that six thousand dollars. The commissioners were also instructed to receive "subscription and donations, for the purpose of erecting suitable buildings and improvements" for the housing and treatment of the insane.[4] Donations for this project must have been slim, indeed, because the 1846 state legislature appropriated a sum of fifteen thousand dollars to erect the "Indiana Hospital for the Insane" on the grounds of the land previously purchased. This act also authorized the previously appointed board of commissioners to appoint a superintendent.[5] This first hospital was located on the west side of Indianapolis and eventually was renamed Central State Hospital.

In 1855 the Indiana General Assembly passed "An act to provide for the confinement of persons insane and dangerous when suffered to run at large and for the compensation of him to whom the custody of such insane person is committed." This act provided that a complaint could be made to a justice of the peace about the sanity of a person and that the justice could issue a warrant for the sheriff to apprehend this person. Subsequently a jury of six householders in the county were to be convened to judge whether the person was insane or not. If insane, a person could be chosen to confine the insane individual or the person could be sent to the hospital for the insane. If the insane person's estate was worth more than five hundred dollars, the person's estate could be assessed to help pay for the confinement and treatment. If the person was not found insane, court charges could be assessed against the complaining party.[6] This law appears to be the first in Indiana to specify a criterion (dangerousness) for commitment to a state mental health facility, or to make provisions to protect the suspected ill person from specious charges.

In 1881 the Indiana General Assembly passed "An act regulating sanity inquests, and the committal of insane persons to hospitals for the insane, and their discharge therefrom." This act provided questions to be asked of the complaining party at the insanity inquest. These twenty-two questions asked for information on name, address, relationship to complaining party, age, height, weight, birthplace, occupation, hair color, marriage duration, number of children, emotional and behavioral symptoms ("talkative, noisy, violent, sleepless, profane, obscene, restless, destructive, homicidal, suicidal, filthy, cheerful, silent melancholy, quiet, seclusive, dull, epileptic, syphilitic, scrofulous, phthisical, hysterical, choretic, deformed, criminal, intemperate, deaf, mute, blind, lame, or paralyzed." "delusions" or "moral deficiencies."), previous hospitalizations, evidence of physical injury, medical history, family history, emotional precipitants ("mental shock or strain"), "indulgence in venereal excess," need for restraint, value of the estate, and use of "opium or chloral" [hydrate]. A form was provided for the examining physician to complete. If the person was judged insane at the insanity inquest, the justice of the peace signed a certificate, which was filed with the clerk of the county's circuit court. The clerk of the circuit court then had to apply to the Indiana Hospital for the Insane for admission. The superintendent had to admit the patient if the case was deemed recent and curable. If the case was not recent or deemed incurable, the insane person could be admitted if space was available. "Idiots," or those with "feeblemindedness," could not be admitted. If the person was accepted for admission, the clerk was to direct the county sheriff or another suitable person to bring the individual to the hospital. The clerk was also directed to procure necessary clothing for the person to be confined.[7]

In 1883 the Indiana General Assembly passed "An act providing for the location of additional hospitals for the insane, and providing management thereof."[8] This act provided for the appointment of a board of commissioners who were "to superintend the location, the letting, the construction, and the equipping of three [additional] hospitals for the insane; and that none of said hospitals shall be erected within fifty miles of the city of Indianapolis." In 1889 the 1883 act was amended in order to designate which Indiana counties could send persons to which hospital (Central Hospital for the Insane, Southern Hospital for the Insane, Eastern Hospital for the Insane, or Northern Hospital for the Insane).[9]

In 1905 the Indiana General Assembly passed "An act concerning the disposition and custody of persons who become insane after conviction for crime, providing how such insanity shall be determined, and providing by whom the costs and expenses of such proceeding may be paid." This act provided that if a convicted defendant appeared to be insane, a jury of twelve was to be impaneled by the court. If the jury found the individual insane, then the defendant could be confined in a "state insane hospital."[10]

In 1909 the Indiana General Assembly passed "An act authorizing and providing for the establishment of a hospital for insane criminals" as a part of the 'Indiana State Prison,' making appropriations therefore, providing for its government and maintenance, defining the manner of holding insanity inquests in cases of conviction alleged to be insane and for their transfer or discharge, repealing all laws in conflict and declaring an emergency." This act appropriated sixty-five thousand dollars to build a hospital for insane criminals within the confines of the Indiana State Prison at Michigan City. The new hospital was to contain 145 beds and, of course, was to treat only "male insane criminals." Any insane convicts housed in any of the state mental hospitals were to be transferred to this new hospital upon completion. This act also provided that those defendants who had been judged not guilty by reason of insanity should be confined in this new hospital.[11]

In 1927 the Indiana General Assembly passed "An act to rename the hospitals for the insane, prescribing the rights, powers and duties of such hospitals as a result of the change in the names and providing for the conclusion of proceedings begun under or by the name by which such hospitals were formerly known." This act provided for the renaming of Indiana's state "hospitals for the insane." The four state hospitals then in existence were to be renamed, Central State Hospital, Richmond State Hospital, Logansport State Hospital, and Evansville State Hospital.[12]

In 1945 the Indiana General Assembly passed an act to create a teaching hospital on the Indiana University Medical Center campus in Indianapolis. This hospital was "to be made available for instruction of medical students, student nurses, interns and resident physicians under the supervision of the faculty of the Indiana University School of Medicine for use by said school in connection with research and instruction in psychiatric disorders."[13] This act created the hospital later named for Dr. Larue D. Carter.

The "criminal sexual psychopathic person" law was passed in 1949.[14] This law defined a criminal sexual psychopathic person as "any person over the age of sixteen years who is suffering from a mental disorder and is not insane or feebleminded, which mental disorder is coupled with criminal propensities to the commission of sex offenses, is hereby declared to be a criminal sexual psychopathic person." This particular law cast a broad net over such offenses, but never really defined what it was, except that it was not murder, manslaughter, or rape of a female child under age twelve. The law provided that the prosecutor file a statement with the court charging such an offense and then the court was to appoint two physicians to examine the individual and make a report with the court. If both agreed that the person was a criminal sexual psychopathic person then a hearing would take place with the judge as to whether that condition existed. If indeed the person was adjudged a criminal sexual psychopathic person, then that person was to be committed to the Council of Mental Health who would then place the person in an appropriate state institution for treatment. No trial was to be held if the person was adjudged to be a criminal sexual psychopathic person.

The decade from 1955-65 saw a number of new mental health laws. In 1955 a law was passed "prescribing the procedure for the restoration of civil rights of patients who are discharged from psychiatric hospitals."[15] This law required the hospital superintendent to report to the court when a committed patient was discharged. The only problem was that some circuit courts ignored the law and never restored a patient's rights to marry, enter into contracts, etc. Eventually Indiana passed a law whereby civil rights were not taken away when a patient was committed to a hospital. In 1965, the Indiana General Assembly passed a law defining a "mentally ill person" and specifically defining "voluntary admission," "temporary commitment," and regular commitment" for the first time.[16]

Since 1970 the number of Indiana laws dealing with mental health issues has skyrocketed. Such laws have included provision for the remuneration of work done in state hospitals (1971), patients' rights (1973, 1979), repeal of sterilization laws (1974) (See next section of this chapter), revision of criminal insanity (1977, 1978, 1980), access to health records (1982), information given to family members (1985), living wills (1985), revision of commitment laws (1987, 1988), and the closing of Central State Hospital and the state developmental facilities.

## Eugenics

In retrospect, the story of eugenics in Indiana and elsewhere in the United States is a particularly sorry chapter for psychiatry. Indiana has the dubious distinction of passing the first eugenics law in 1907. One of the aims of this law was to sterilize "confirmed criminals, idiots, imbeciles and rapists."[1] Nearly thirty other states followed Indiana's lead in passing similar laws. However, starting with Governor Thomas Marshall, several Indiana governors ignored implementation of the law until it was ruled unconstitutional by the Indiana Supreme Court in 1921.

In 1915 Governor Samuel Ralston appointed a Committee of Mental Defectives at the State Board of Charities. The charge to the committee was "to study the serious problem of the state's epileptic, feebleminded, and insane and decide how to fight mental defectiveness, the most important cause of pauperism, degeneracy and crime in Indiana."[1-2] The members of this committee included Samuel E. Smith, M.D., superintendent of the Eastern Indiana Hospital for the Insane and Mary A. Spink, M.D., former employee of the Indiana Hospital for the Insane and medical superintendent of Neuronhurst. Over the next several years the committee and its hired field workers collected data from several Indiana counties and found that two percent of Indiana's population was mentally defective. In one of the committee's studies[3] Putnam County was found to have "sheltered for many years a class of people listless, lazy and indifferent. These people have intermarried because of geographical features of the county about them and have intermingled little with the more intelligent and mentally active people of the rich lands at the north of the county."

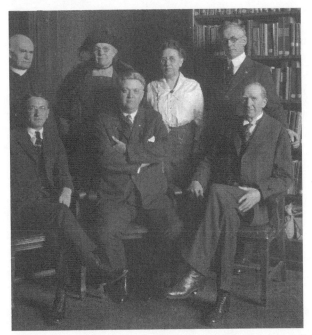

Indiana State Board of Charities, October 1920; seated left to right are Rabbi M.M. Feuerlich, Rev. L.A. Harrison, and Amos W. Butler; standing left to right are Francis H. Govisk, Sarah A. Dinwiddie, Mary A. Spink, M.D., and William J. Sayers.
Photo courtesy of Indiana State Archives, Commission
on Public Records. All rights reserved.

Ultimately the committee's work resulted in the passage of a second sterilization law in 1927.[4] This law provided for the sterilization of "any such patient confined in any such institution afflicted with hereditary forms of insanity that are recurrent, idiocy, imbecility, feeblemindedness or epilepsy." Such individuals could come from "any hospital or other institution of the state, or any county of the state, which has the care or custody" of these individuals. All that was required to carry out this law was a petition, hearing, and order of the county circuit court.

Over the succeeding years nearly 2,424 sterilizations of "mental defectives" were carried out in Indiana until the law was repealed in 1974 under Governor Ortis Bowen, M.D.[3] This number included 1,167 men and 1,257 women. One thousand seven hundred and fifty-one were mentally deficient and 677 mentally ill. Most of these sterilizations occurred before 1955. About eighteen hundred sterilizations were performed by the Fort Wayne School for Feebleminded Youth. Other sterilizations were performed at Muscatatuck, Logansport State Hospital, Indiana Girls School and the Indiana State Reformatory.[5-6]

## Preliminary Mental Examination

Between the years of 1967-75 many patients were admitted to Marion County General Hospital (later renamed Wishard Hospital) on what was called a "pre-mental exam" or preliminary mental examination. This type of involuntary hospitalization was only used in Indianapolis at General Hospital. The pre-mental exam allowed the hospital to hold an involuntary psychiatric patient for up to ten days while his or her behavior was observed by doctors and other hospital personnel. If the patient did not fit the criteria for a temporary commitment then he or she was released. If, on the other hand, the patient did meet criteria for a temporary commitment, then the appropriate paperwork was filed with the court to initiate proceedings for a commitment.

The preliminary mental examination was established in 1945 by the Indiana General Assembly.[1] This law was passed for persons who were suspected of "insanity" but who refused to be examined by a physician so that the commitment process could be initiated through a prior 1927 law governing commitments. This law allowed any "reputable citizen" of a county to swear out an affidavit stating that he or she believed a person to be insane. The affidavit was then presented to the "superintendent of the psychopathic ward of the city hospital of any city of the first class."

If approved by the superintendent, the affidavit was to be filed with the municipal court clerk and presented to a judge for further action. The judge could then issue a "writ of detention" for that person allowing the person to be detained in the hospital for a period of ten days. The writ could be extended for a further period of time based upon the recommendation of the superintendent. The writ was then given to the police and the person was picked up and transported to the hospital for examination. A reasonable amount of bail was allowed. In addition the law allowed for a stay of trial in cases of criminal charges. Persons could be temporarily held in the county jail if there was no room in the hospital. The superintendent could also approve transfer to a private hospital or a veterans' hospital. When the Indiana General Assembly finally passed a law allowing for an immediate detention and a seventy-two hour hold, this law was no longer necessary.

## Mental Health Court: Indiana's Most Unique Court[1]

The time for the commitment hearing has come and a patient and hospital attendant are on their way to court. The elevator doors open on a small vestibule marked Marion County Municipal Court Three. Turning down the carpeted hall they enter the small courtroom, replete with oak bench, brass rail, counselor's tables and microphones. Not only was this court solely for mental health cases, its location was also quite unique: it was inside Wishard Hospital, two floors above the psychiatric unit.

In 1980 the court was started to help divert the mentally ill from the criminal justice system and into the mental health system for appropriate treatment. This allowed persons arrested on a Disorderly Conduct Question Mark (DOC?) charge (applied to disorderly people about whose sanity the officer had questions) to be brought directly to the Wishard Hospital emergency room rather than taken directly to jail. In the emergency room, staffed with police to ensure custody, the patient was assessed by physicians and workers from Midtown Mental Health Center. Persons needing hospitalization could be admitted from the emergency room.

Prior to 1980, these cases were seen by fourteen courts with fourteen different judges. Patients who were admitted directly to the hospital usually had their charges dropped without a court appearance and were often unaware that their behavior was a community concern. Midtown Community Mental Health Center opened negotiations with Probate Court Judge Evan Goodman who had developed a keen interest in the problems of the mentally ill and close working relationship with court psychiatrists. Plans for the court emerged. The hospital allocated the space and the mental health center funded a full-time clinical position for liaison to the court. The court liaison met with patients and family members to help them get started in treatment and to educate them about the charges or commitment. A psychiatrist was assigned each day for occasional pre-court re-evaluations.

The response from patients and the community was very positive and in January 1982 the court was made permanent through state legislative action. In May 1985, the DOC? was challenged and declared illegal. Since then, people have been slated into court on other misdemeanor charges (public intoxication, disorderly conduct, trespassing, etc). Some defendants were sent to jail from the emergency room, some were admitted and a few were released on their own recognizance. Patients charged with felonies were seen in other courts.

Judge Goodman developed a unique courtroom style that combined law and common sense advice. Patients were expected to follow through with the court-ordered treatment and present a progress report from their therapist. Under the DOC? charge, patients who did not follow the court's orders, could be transferred to another court for trial, be charged with contempt of court, or face up to one hundred eighty days in jail. Favorable reports resulted in Judge Goodman praising patients' successes and occasionally even taking them to lunch. His flexible style resulted in the court occasionally meeting in the intensive care unit when a suicidal patient was unable to come to court personally.

Dr. Elizabeth Bowman interviewed Judge Goodman about his experiences in this unique court. The following excerpt from that interview conveys some of the practical and compassionate tone he brought to this court.

Dr. Bowman:     "How did this court get started?"

Judge Goodman: "In 1980 this court began as a pilot project because the Indianapolis Bar Association, the Municipal Court System, Midtown Community Mental Health Center, lawyers and judges were interested in getting the DOC? cases out of the municipal courts. Most municipal judges didn't know how to deal with them, didn't want them and certainly didn't think that some guy who was naked directing traffic was very important compared to rape or murder cases. People who were taken to Wishard were not coming to court and those who were seen in court were simply taken to jail and not given any workup. More often than not if a DOC? went to a downtown court the judge would say it was not really a crime and would dismiss the case. There would be no follow-up and no one would go to treatment, so we decided to try the court at the hospital.

Dr. Bowman: "Were there other reasons for the court?"

Judge Goodman: "Protecting patient rights was another reason for having this court. Before 1976 physicians almost never went to court. Mrs. Hill, the liaison person between the hospital and the court would get the clinical information from the hospital mental health worker hospital, go to all the municipal courts and tell the judges what the doctor found. A bond would be set, the patient would be secured in Wishard and patients almost never got to see a court or have their rights protected. The judges would sign orders based on Mrs. Hill's report of what the doctor said. The judges wouldn't have known a psychosis if one bit them so they would renew Preliminary Mental Exam orders for another 10 days ad nauseum without the patient going to court. Patients get better care since we have more consistency of treatment with one court instead of fourteen. Here we have all kinds of experts available."

Dr. Bowman: "What kinds of cases do you see?"

Judge Goodman: "In the beginning we were not a full-time court and saw only DOC? and PME cases. Under the pilot project I was a full-time lawyer coming here on my lunch hour to hear cases. The Probate Court still had exclusive jurisdiction over civil commitments. The legislature made this a full-time court in 1982 Initially we ran seven sessions a week here and three in an outlying traffic court until we got enough business that we quit doing the traffic court. Now we see commitments, domestic cases PME's and Emergency Detentions".

Dr. Bowman: "Why was this court called the "Basketball Court?"

Judge Goodman: "Initially we used a room that was a mental health patient recreation area and there was a basketball goal over the bench. The patients waited in the kitchenette at the back of the courtroom behind a big glass door and we would just motion to them when it was their turn. We made a bench of tables disguised by a tablecloth. We finally got to the place where we had a rollaway bench that we stored in the kitchenette with our eclectic collection of chairs. The patients used the room during the day and at noon we would roll out the bench and hold what we called 'the Castor Court.'"

Dr. Bowman: "Now you have a beautiful court room, two bailiffs, a recorder and a clerk. Do you think this court is cost efficient?"

Judge Goodman: "I have no question but that this has saved millions of dollars. If the average alcoholic spends $146,000 in his/her lifetime on alcohol and if you can encourage this person to stop drinking you may prevent all the police runs, all the beatings and all the stupidities that occur because someone is abusing alcohol. It seems that once or twice through this court often makes a difference. If someone gets a GED or is offered an opportunity to be a creative productive citizen instead of abusing the resources of the community, there is no way to calculate the savings."

Dr. Bowman: "What are the advantages of having a mental health court?"

Judge Goodman: "The expertise that is gathered, the convenience, and the consistent treatment of all people in one court. I generally know when a doctor knows his or her field and I am not intimidated by medical jargon. "Most judges automatically believe a doctor who says a patient is sick. The patient may very well be sick but the test is whether that illness impairs the person's ability to function. We all may be sick in some way, but we all have to fit in our community".

Dr. Bowman: "What were physicians' initial reactions to the court?"

Judge Goodman: "Initially some were quite incensed that anyone was going to tell them what to do with their patients. The law changed in 1976, requiring doctors to be present for civil commitments unless that right was waived by the patient. Now when a patient refuses therapy, doctors have to decide how serious they are about wanting the patient in the hospital. If the doctor doesn't want to go to court, the patient is given a choice about treatment with that doctor. So the very system being in place probably helps patient rights and informed consent."

Dr. Bowman: "How did you come to be the judge of this court?"

Judge Goodman: "I was working one day a week as civil commitment commissioner in the probate court. I was the last commissioner hired so I got stuck with the new commitment load. I went to Muscatatuck State Hospital to hold hearings I found that the aquatic therapy pool was an important treatment for a bedfast patient but the pool was broken and he hadn't been treated for six months. I ordered the pool fixed. Neither the hospital nor I knew a commissioner didn't have the authority to do that, so they fixed it. At that moment I realized I could do something for people that nobody seemed to care about."

Dr. Bowman: "I had one hospitalized patient who was arrested on a DOC?. At her hearing you read her the riot act and it had a tremendous impact on her. During the entire hospitalization she lived in fear that you would put her in jail if she didn't comply with treatment. She disappeared the minute her charges were dropped. You have been known to give advice to patients from the bench. What is your reason for doing that?"

Judge Goodman: It may be that I think I can get away with saying things that a psychiatrist can't say because I am wearing the robes. I think I offer people an opportunity to fit in. I do whatever I can to see that they take advantage of that opportunity, whether I am offering a battered woman a powerful ally in her marriage or encouraging people to use their potential more. The goal is not to make people think alike but to see that they don't disrupt the community. There's no law against suicide in Indiana but when manipulative suicidal behavior jeopardizes innocent people as happens when a suicidal patient turns on the gas in an apartment and jeopardizes everyone else in the building, then that's not fair. Unless somebody makes a patient look at that behavior, the law is not doing its job. In offering an opportunity to protect people's rights, I am not just interested in the defendant's rights. The community has a right to be safe from people who will jeopardize it."

Dr. Bowman: "What do psychiatrists do in court that really bothers you?"

Judge Goodman: "Not being prepared for their case really bugs me. I have to look to the psychiatrist to give me direction and guidance in what I am going to do with that case. Unless they are well prepared, they might as well not come to court. There have been times when I had to recess cases and give the doctor time to go back and figure out the diagnosis, what the case is all about and what medications the patient is on. Sometimes I have dismissed cases because of inadequate evidence from the doctor. If the doctor had been prepared, she or he could have done a good job for the patient but if the doctors don't know what is going on, how do they expect me to know?"

Dr. Bowman: "What do you think psychiatry residents should be taught about coming into court and testifying?"

Judge Goodman: "That they shouldn't be afraid of courts, that court can be part of the therapeutic process and how they can be therapeutic in court. Being honest and not pulling punches is one of the best things they can do. I've seen how the court is used therapeutically in the DOC? cases. When a person has been arrested on a DOC? And becomes an outpatient without a civil commitment, in return for the prosecutor withholding prosecution for disorderly conduct, then that person needs to go and find out why she disrupted the community. If she comes back with a positive report from the clinic, the case will be dismissed. If not, then she is looking at one hundred eighty days. When patients bring back reports that say they showed up and worked hard, I read the letters to them and it is part of the therapeutic process to have a powerful judge applaud how well they did. Psychiatrists also need to learn not to take court cases so personally. You are not the ones on trial. Whether you win or lose the case is not as important as offering your patients chances to do things differently and get some wisdom in their behavior. If they avail themselves of that, you have done something therapeutic. Psychiatrists can also do much more with the families of schizophrenics without breaching privileged communications. It makes no sense to make someone well and then send them back into an environment that helped make them sick. Urge families to go to support groups or Al-Anon. Even if the patient does not get well, the family can avoid being manipulated. Talking to families from the bench is a major part of what goes on here, as is treating everyone with dignity even when I'm tired and they are the dregs of humanity.

Dr. Bowman:    "Why was the DOC? was declared illegal?"

Judge Goodman:    "It didn't offer enough rights. Last year I proposed a reckless endangerment law that was constitutional and offered rights, but it did not pass the legislature. Right now we have Immediate Detention, a twenty-four hour hold. The problem is that patients don't have to go to court and are not held accountable for destructive behavior. I think what made this court so successful is that people knew they had to come back and face the same judge. Like the lady you mentioned, she was gone as soon as she knew she was out from under the gun. Dr. Alan Schmetzer and others did a study that found the rearrest rate of chronically mentally ill patients who came through this court on the DOC? was quite low. This tells me that whatever happened in this court worked.

Dr. Bowman:    "What was your most unusual case?"

Judge Goodman:    "My most exciting case was a lawyer from another state who became psychotic and was arrested on a DOC?. He came to court in his hospital gown and strutted down the aisle holding forth like he was in front of the jury. To keep him from taking control of the court I asked him if he knew about Satre and told him that I could imagine him standing there like Satre would, wondering why the rest of the world thinks he is crazy but really knowing that they are the ones who are out of touch. That struck a chord in him and we began to discuss Satre. Finally, some drunk in the back of the room belched and broke our concentration. I looked up and there was this entire courtroom just gawking at us, probably not understanding anything we said. Someone suggested to me later that I had gotten into his psychosis. I had never heard of that. I just thought that I met people where they are."

The mental health court no longer resides at Wishard Hospital since it was dissolved in the early 1990s. Currently civil commitments in Marion County, Indiana are handled by the Probate Division of Marion County Civil Court Eight. Marion County Criminal Court Eight handles many of the minor crimes committed by mentally ill persons. Court Eight places some seriously and chronically mentally ill defendants who are charged with minor crimes into a mental health diversion program known as the PAIR (Psychiatric Assertive Identification and Referral) program. This program works in cooperation with the Marion County Prosecutor's Office, Marion County Public Defender's Office, Marion County Superior Court, and the community mental health centers serving Marion County.

## Landmark Indiana Cases

Landmark court decisions are court decisions which establish legal precedents or often establish new legal principals or concepts. Landmark decisions often change or advance the interpretation of existing case law. Many such cases involve the Supreme Court of the United States. Indiana has had its share of landmark decisions, of which this chapter describes a selected few. All material selected for inclusion here came from public sources such as newspaper and magazine articles, legal citations, and professional legal and medical articles.

## Jackson v Indiana[1]

Theon Jackson was a mentally retarded deaf mute man living in Marion County, Indiana. He was unable to read or write and could only communicate through very limited sign language. In July 1967 he snatched a purse containing four dollars and a short time later snatched another purse containing five dollars. He entered a plea of not guilty in the criminal court system in Marion County, Indiana. Since his competence to stand trial was questioned, two court-appointed psychiatrists examined Mr. Jackson. Both physicians opined that Jackson was incompetent to stand trial because of his various deficiencies. Neither psychiatrist was hopeful that Mr. Jackson could be restored to competency. Based upon the psychiatrists' examinations, the court ruled Jackson incompetent to stand trial and ordered him committed to the Indiana Department of Mental Health for restoration of competency to stand trial. Mr. Jackson's attorney filed an appeal with the court and argued that since he was not insane and could not be restored to competency that Mr. Jackson had received, in effect, a life sentence to a mental institution for a petty crime. The trial court denied the appeal as did the Indiana Supreme court with one judge dissenting.

The United States Supreme court granted certiorari. Upon hearing the case, the Court reversed the decision of the Indiana Supreme Court. The justices held that Indiana could not indefinitely commit Mr. Jackson because he was incompetent to stand trial. This, they reasoned, violated the equal protection and due process clauses of the Fourteenth Amendment. The court also ruled that if there was not a substantial probability that Jackson could obtain competency to stand trial, then the state must institute civil commitment proceedings or release him.

## Burns v Reed[2]

On September 2, 1982 Cathy Burns called the Muncie, Indiana Police Department and reported that an unknown assailant had shot her two young sons after they had knocked her unconscious. Two Muncie police officers were assigned to her case. They came to view her as the primary suspect even though she had passed a lie detector test and voice stress analysis and had repeatedly denied shooting her sons. The officers suspected that Burns might have multiple personality and wanted her interviewed during hypnosis. Prior to having her hypnotized, however, they sought the advice of chief deputy prosecutor, Richard Reed. Reed advised them to go ahead. Burns was hypnotized by a hired hypnotist and while in a hypnotic trance she referred to the assailant as "Katie," another part of herself. At the probable cause hearing the judge was told that the "suspect" had confessed but the judge was not informed that the "confession" was obtained under hypnosis. Burns was charged with attempted murder but her confession was suppressed since it was obtained during hypnosis. The charges were dropped against Burns. In 1985 Burns filed an action in the United States District Court for the Southern District of Indiana against the police officers and prosecutor. Although the police officers settled out of court, the action proceeded to trial against defendant Reed. The court granted Reed a directed verdict by finding that Reed was immune from liability because he was acting in his official duties as a prosecutor. When taken to the United States Supreme Court, the justices held that Reed was absolutely immune from civil damages based upon his initiating a prosecution and presenting the state's case. However, they also held that Reed was not immune from civil damages caused by his offering advice to the police and that the civil case could proceed.

### Indiana v Edwards[3-5]

In July 1999 Ahmad Edwards was in the process of stealing a pair of shoes from an Indianapolis, Indiana department store. He was discovered in the act, fired a gun at a security officer, and then shot and wounded a bystander. He was charged with theft, attempted murder, battery with a deadly weapon, and criminal recklessness.

Over the next three years Edwards was the subject of three competency to stand trial proceedings (August 2000, March 2002, and April 2003). At the first competency hearing Edwards was found incompetent to stand trial and sent to Logansport State Hospital for restoration of competency. Seven months after he was hospitalized the hospital's physicians found Edwards competent to stand trial. After he returned to jail, his attorney asked for another competency evaluation, but this time after considering additional evidence, Edwards was again found competent to stand trial. Seven months later Edward's attorney asked for yet another competency examination. After further psychiatric examinations Edwards was found incompetent to stand trial and sent back to Logansport State Hospital. Eight months later in June 2005 hospital physicians again found Edwards competent to stand trial.

Edwards' trial began in 2006 and at that time he asked to represent himself. After the court refused his request, the trial continued, and Edwards was convicted of criminal recklessness and theft, but the jury was unable to reach a verdict on the other more serious charges of battery and attempted murder. Because of this, the state decided to retry Edwards on the remaining charges. Edwards again requested to represent himself. The court refused his request, however, and reasoned that although he had schizophrenia and was competent to stand trial, he was not competent to defend himself. The trial went forward and Edwards was convicted on the remaining two counts. He was sentenced to thirty years in jail.

Edwards appealed his conviction to the Indiana Appellate Court and argued that the trial court had denied him his constitutional right of self-representation. Edwards won his appeal and the court ordered a new trial. The matter then landed in the Indiana Supreme Court who agreed with the Indiana Appellate Court. The case was then appealed to the United States Supreme Court. Prior to the United States Supreme Court hearing the matter, nineteen states, the American Bar Association, the American Psychiatric Association, and the American Academy of Psychiatry and the Law filed amicus briefs which supported Indiana in requiring a higher standard for competency to represent oneself.

The Supreme Court ruled that, in essence, competency to stand trial and competency to represent one's self were two different issues with two different sets of criteria, although the court did not specifically outline the standards for competency to represent oneself. The court indicated that competency to represent oneself required a higher standard than competency to stand trial since an attorney represents the defendant if one is found competent to stand trial.

## Chapter 16

# Cases, Famous and Infamous

County Clerk: "What's your name?"
John Zwara: "I don't know."
County Clerk: "What's your mother's name?"
John Zwara: "I don't know."
County Clerk: "At what port did you land when you came to this country?"
John Zwara: "I don't know – maybe Omaha."

> As told by Alexander Vonnegut,
> in Charles S. Bonsett. John Zwara.
> *Indiana Medical History Quarterly*, 1 (1),
> July, 1973, p. 3.

In researching for this book we have come across some interesting psychiatric cases. What follows are five fascinating cases, two from the nineteenth century and three from the twentieth century. The material from all five of these cases is drawn from previously published accounts in books, newspapers, and magazines. No case patient records were utilized.

### Anna Keyt Agnew

Anna Keyt Agnew was born in Ohio in 1836. In her book, *From Under the Cloud*, she dated the onset of her illness to precisely November 19, 1876.[1] Looking back at age 50, Anna described herself as having been born with a "suicidal tendency" and having had a "depressed temperament since childhood." She described her childhood personality as "proud, willful, and not always obedient." At the onset of her illness Anna was married and had three sons. Overnight she descended into depression, "a dreadful place of darkness." She made several suicide attempts by hanging and poisoning with laudanum, chloral hydrate, "sugar of lead," and strychnine.

Ultimately her husband and physician had her committed from their home in Vincennes, Indiana to the Indiana Hospital for the Insane in Indianapolis. Anna was to remain in the hospital for the next seven years. She wrote her book in 1886 to bring attention to the abuses which occurred in state hospitals.

Anna's writing style is lively and tends towards the dramatic. She is not afraid to call a spade a spade. She lavishes praise on some of her several doctors and a few kindly attendants. Some of the attendants, however, she described as sadistic rulers of the individual fiefdoms or wards in which they worked. If one didn't immediately follow their orders to go to the dining room and eat or retire to bed, patients got dragged to the dining room and force fed or dragged off to bed and restrained. Anna wrote with some satisfaction when the new superintendent, Dr. Fletcher, abolished the use of restraints and burned them all in a Christmas bonfire (See chapter 2).

Anna's periods of depression were broken by periods of manic excitement which were characterized by laughing, praying, and delusions about Masonry. She once spent a year on the epileptic ward, although she described no signs of epilepsy in her book. In her book, *The seven steeples: Anna Agnew and the Indiana Hospital for the Insane*, psychiatrist Lucy Jane King, M.D., correctly diagnosed Mrs. Agnew as suffering from bipolar disorder.[2]

During Anna's hospitalization, through no fault of her own, she became estranged from her husband, David Agnew. He was a sometimes visitor and at his last visit with Anna in 1883 he claimed exclusive ownership of their children. She bitingly suggested that he "take out a patent" on this "novel" idea. On discharge from the hospital she went to Aurora, Indiana where her children were living. She ultimately dedicated her book, which she wrote from Pittsburg, Pennsylvania, to her children.

While at the hospital Anna became addicted to chloral hydrate, a sedative prescribed for sleep. Although she liked most of her physicians, who included Drs. Harris, Rogers, Thomas, and Stockton, she disliked assistant physician Dr. John C. Walker, who punitively withheld her chloral hydrate prompting her to go into withdrawal.[3]

While at the Indiana Hospital for the Insane, Anna worked a year in the sewing room before she was discharged in April, 1885. Her descriptions of other patients showed a keen sense of observation and penetrating insight. A number of patients had delusions of being famous personages of the time, such as Mrs. President Hayes or Mrs. Ex-President Arthur.

One of the most interesting patents was "Auntie H," or the "autocrat of the dining room." Auntie H believed that she was being paid eighty million dollars a year to be superintendent of the universe. She believed that she had been married seventeen times and that she had two hundred fifty children. She also apparently talked incessantly from sunup to sundown. Auntie H was likely another well-described example of bipolar disorder.

## Anthony G. Kiritsis[1-5]

On the morning of February 8, 1977 former used-car salesman Anthony G. "Tony" Kiritis arrived at the Market Street office of Meridian Mortgage Company President Richard O. Hall in downtown Indianapolis and took Mr. Hall hostage. Mr. Kiritsis pulled a sawed-off shotgun out of a long flower box and wired it to Mr. Hall's neck with a coat-hanger wire. This "dead man's line" meant that if the police shot Mr. Kiritsis, his weight would pull the trigger on the shotgun and kill Mr. Hall. Prior to parading Mr. Hall through several downtown Indianapolis streets, Mr. Kiritsis, clad in a short-sleeved shirt in below-freezing temperatures, called the police. Near the State Capital Building Kiritsis commandeered a police car and forced Hall to drive him to his Crestwood Village West apartment on the west side of town. Once inside the apartment Kiritsis claimed that his apartment was rigged with explosives. Thus began a harrowing 63-hour, three-day standoff with the police.

Prior to this dramatic hostage-taking incident, Mr. Kiritsis had fallen behind on a one hundred thirty thousand dollar mortgage on a seventeen-acre property on the west side of Indianapolis where he was planning to build a strip mall. Mr. Hall, the mortgage broker, had repeatedly given Mr. Kiritsis additional time to make payments but time had run out. Mr. Kiritsis became convinced that Hall's company had steered buyers for the property away so that Hall's company could make more money on the considerably appreciated land.

During the time that Mr. Hall was being held hostage, Mr. Kiritsis made calls to the news media, including radio and television stations. WIBC Radio talk-show host Fred Heckman actually broadcast some of their decidedly one-sided conversations that were strongly laced with profanities.

Marion County Sheriff's detective Sgt. Ronald Beasley indicated that he had arrested Mr. Kiritsis several years previously on a malicious trespass complaint filed by a relative. In addition he said, "He's a very hot tempered individual…When he gets mad he does just about anything he wants to."[6] A previous arrest included a charge of assault with intent to murder in 1968. Mr. Kiritsis had also been arrested after firing shots at his brother about twelve years prior to the hostage taking incident.[7]

Mr. Kiritsis finally released Hall after the Meridian Mortgage Company promised to cancel the loan, say that they had mistreated Mr. Kiritsis, and pay him five million dollars. Prosecutors also promised not to prosecute Mr. Kiritsis. After releasing Hall, Kiritsis fired his shotgun in order to prove that it had been loaded. However, no explosives were found in Kiritsis' apartment.

About a year after Kiritsis was captured, he was tried for kidnapping, armed extortion, and armed robbery in Marion County Superior Court Five. Nile Stanton was chief defense counsel and J. Richard Kiefer was co-counsel. The prosecutors included F. Thomas Schornhorst and George Montgomery. The trial judge was the Honorable Michael Dugan. Although Mr. Kiritsis did not want to use an insanity defense, he reluctantly agreed to use it on advice of counsel.

At the time of the trial the burden of proof, when an insanity case was tried, was on the state to prove sanity beyond a reasonable doubt. During the jury selection, Judge Dugan did not allow the defense or prosecution ask the prospective jurors questions. Judge Dugan asked questions himself using questions submitted by both defense and prosecution.

During the trial a number of psychiatrists gave conflicting testimony as to the mental state of Mr. Kiritsis at the time of the alleged crime. Iver Small, M.D., one of the three court-ordered psychiatrists appointed to examine Mr. Kiritsis, opined that Mr. Kiritsis was suffering from a mental disease or defect at the time of the alleged crime so that he could not conform his conduct to the requirements of the law. Both Dr. Small and the defense psychiatrist, Larry Davis, M.D., opined that Mr. Kiritsis was suffering from a "paranoid delusional" disorder. Mr. Kiritsis took the stand and testified in his own defense. His attorney, Nile Stanton, believed Kiritsis did an incredible job. The defense also put on a number of witnesses who testified that he was a good person and couldn't have been in his right mind when he took Mr. Hall hostage.

After a two-week trial and thirty-five hours of jury deliberation, Mr. Kiritsis was found not guilty by reason of insanity (NGRI). His acquittal and the acquittal of John Hinkley, the man who shot then-President Ronald Reagan, prompted Indiana legislators to change the NGRI law in Indiana. Henceforth, the burden of proof would be on the defendant to prove insanity and the criteria for insanity was changed to requiring that the defendant have a pervasive mental disease or defect causing him or her not to be able to understand the wrongfulness of their conduct at the time of the commission of the alleged crime.

After his conviction in late 1977, Mr. Kiritsis was remanded to the custody of the police. What followed was a bizarre saga through several mental health and correctional institutions until Kiritsis was finally released from Central State Hospital in January 1988. Mr. Kiritsis was initially taken to Larue D. Carter Memorial Hospital where he stayed from November 1977 until March of 1980 when he was transferred to Logansport State Hospital after a commitment hearing was held. During his time at Logansport State Hospital he was transferred temporarily to the Pendleton Reformatory because he continued to refuse to undergo a psychiatric examination so physicians could formulate a treatment plan.

During his hospitalization at Carter Hospital Mr. Kiritsis, through his attorney Richard Kiefer, filed a petition for a writ of mandate and prohibition with the Indiana Supreme Court. At the time Mr. Kiritsis was being held in contempt of the Marion County Probate Court for failure to cooperate and undergo a psychiatric examination. The Supreme Court denied the petition. In its opinion, the court held that the privilege against self-incrimination had no applicability in this case since a civil commitment was not a criminal proceeding.[8]

In December 1984 Madison County Superior Court Judge Dennis Carroll refused to lift the contempt of court charge against Mr. Kiritsis, who was then being held at the Pendleton Reformatory in Madison County. His attorney, Mr. Stanton, had argued that he should be released because he had been held in contempt of court longer than anyone in Indiana history.[9]

In December 1987, after hearing conflicting testimony from several different psychiatrists, special Judge James E. Harris of the Morgan County Circuit Court opined that the state had failed to prove that Mr. Kiritsis posed a danger to himself or others and ruled that Mr. Kiritsis could be released from Central State Hospital if he were willing to submit to a guardianship to which Mr. Kiritsis refused.[10] By mid-January 1988, however, Mr. Kiritsis was released from Central State Hospital without a guardianship.[11]

In December 1989 Mr. Kiritsis filed a pro se civil suit in Marion Superior Court Three against virtually everyone, excepting his defense team, who had had contact with him following his acquittal by not guilty by reason of insanity. In his suit Mr. Kiritsis alleged that there had been a conspiracy against him to keep him incarcerated. The defendants in this case numbered about one hundred. All cases were dismissed by special judge John Westhalfer.[12]

Mr. Kiritsis died at his home in Speedway, Indiana on January 28, 2005 at the age of seventy-two.

## Maude Ott[1]

In the Fall 2008 edition of the Indiana Psychiatric Society *Spectrum* I [Coons] described the Evansville State Hospital arson fire of February 9, 1943 and the Indiana's rapid evacuation of patients to other state hospitals.[2] (See Chapter 3.) At least eight individuals died in this fire. Below is the forensic investigation of the most likely suspect in this arson.

Maud Lucas (a.k.a. Aleen Elliott) was employed as a psychiatric attendant at Evansville State Hospital at the time of the fire in 1943. Born in Virginia in 1887, she had married James Ott in early 1944. Both before and after the 1943 fire, Mr. and Mrs. Ott had been employed as attendants at several state hospitals in three states: Richmond State Hospital, Madison State Hospital, and Logansport State Hospital in Indiana, Weston State Hospital in West Virginia and Toledo State Hospital in Ohio.[3]

On Wednesday, February 23, 1944 at around 10:00 PM an arson fire occurred at Logansport State Hospital where Mrs. Ott had been employed since early February. Clifford Williams, M.D., was the hospital superintendent at the time.

The fire started in a ground floor storeroom on a women's ward. Kerosene had been used as an accelerant. This fire was the third suspicious fire that had occurred in four days. The first fire had occurred the previous Sunday afternoon in an unoccupied patient's room on the third floor of the fourth ward building and the second occurred in the personnel quarters in the same building on Tuesday morning, February 22.[4]

After Mrs. Ott blamed other attendants for starting the fire at Logansport State Hospital, the police named her as a suspect and she was taken into custody on February 26th along with her husband James who was suspected as having been an accessory. Investigation revealed that kerosene had also been used to start arson fires at Evansville State Hospital in February, 1943 and the state hospital in Toledo, Ohio in January, 1944 where the Otts had been previously employed. A suspicious fire had also occurred at their home in Birdseye, Indiana in April 1943.

Mr. Ott remarked that "It looked suspicious that fires always seemed to follow her."

Mrs. Ott was jailed at the Cass County Jail where she attempted suicide by taking a bottle of sleeping pills two days later on February 28th.[5-8] She apparently had smuggled the bottle of pills into the jail by hiding it in the lining of her coat. She was hospitalized at Cass County Hospital where she remained in a comatose or semi-comatose condition for about a week. Following her recovery she was placed on the detention ward at Cass County Hospital where she threatened to hang herself the next time that she attempted suicide.

On March 2, 1944, Mrs. Ott's husband James was questioned about the fire at Logansport State Hospital and underwent a lie detector test. He reported that his wife had confessed to him that she had started the fire at Evansville State Hospital in a linen closet because she had discovered a "love nest" where psychiatric attendants were having sex. He said that she had started fires at Toledo State Hospital and Logansport State Hospital in order to get even with attendants. He reported that she had started a fire in their home in order to collect insurance money. Mr. Ott painted a story of moving from hospital to hospital in search of jobs after his wife had become dissatisfied with other personnel and working conditions at each facility.[9-10]

Following her husband's polygraph test and written statement, Mrs. Ott was given a lie detector test and was found to have lied about not starting the fires at Logansport State Hospital, Toledo State Hospital and the fire in her home. Polygraph results were inconclusive about the Evansville State Hospital fire.

As time passed, other details emerged about Maud Ott.[11-12] It was reported that she had been hospitalized twice at state hospitals in West Virginia. She finished high school at age seventeen and at age twenty-two she started nurses training which she continued for twenty-two months. At one time, she had taken the name of Aleen Elliott, an attendant at another psychiatric hospital. From 1928-41 she was in and out of different psychiatric hospitals after having experienced an "epileptic psychosis following an abdominal operation." Over the years she had attempted suicide on at least nine occasions via overdose, drowning, wrist cutting, suffocation, and hanging. She lied to her husband about her true age before she married him.

On March 13, 1944 Mrs. Ott said of her husband's statement, "If Jimmy says it's so, it must be so, but I can't believe it."[13] She eventually admitted to setting fire at her home in an upstairs room by pouring kerosene on old newspapers. On March 14, 1944 Mrs. Ott pleaded guilty to second degree arson and was sentenced to one to ten years at the Indiana Women's Prison in Indianapolis.[14] Later in March she was charged with first degree arson of her Birdseye home.[15] While in the Indianapolis Women's Prison Mrs. Ott became "acutely disturbed secondary to epilepsy" and was transferred on September 6, 1944 to, of all places, Logansport State Hospital. Upon admission she was reported to have said, "Won't Dr. Williams be surprised to see me."[16-17]

Also in March, 1944 Mr. Ott was charged with fraud or conspiracy to collect insurance monies after the fire in their Birdseye, Indiana home in Dubois County.[18] It was he who had accepted and deposited the insurance check covering the fire damage to their home. He pleaded not guilty. The trial was delayed on a number of occasions and I was unable to discover the outcome this charge. The charges of being an accessory to the Logansport State Hospital fire were apparently dropped.

Mrs. Ott died on February 1, 1949 while still a patient at Logansport State Hospital.[19] She was never tried for arson and murder in the Evansville State Hospital fire. Prosecutors were uncertain whether her husband could be compelled to testify even though their marriage was in legal limbo because Mrs. Ott had lied about her identity and age.

## Albert Thayer

Albert Thayer was born in Pickinsville, South Carolina in 1836. His parents moved to Indiana with their nine children and settled near Zionsville. After serving Indiana in the Civil War, Mr. Thayer returned to Boone County where he operated a general store until 1874. Eventually he moved to Massachusetts Avenue in Indianapolis where he operated a coal and wood business. He married Matilda Little by whom he had two children.[1]

Mr. Thayer was admitted to the Indiana Hospital for the Insane in the early 1880s. He wrote at least two pamphlets[2-3] and a number of letters to various Indianapolis newspapers to document the existence of abuses within the hospital.

In 1886 Thayer described a typical hospital ward: "A ward is something over a hundred feet long, with a hall about sixteen feet wide running its full length. The hall is flanked on either side by a row of bedrooms as well as a dining room, bath-room, clothes-room, etc. The bedrooms vary in size, containing one to twelve beds. Each ward accommodates from twenty to twenty-five patients, over who are placed two attendants, who receive each twenty to twenty-two dollars a month and board for their services."[1] The attendants were expected to make beds, clean the ward, set tables for meal time, give medications, take patients out for exercise, and keep order on the ward. When he was on ward E, Mr. Thayer observed the attendants slapping, beating, choking, and cursing other patients in order to keep them under control without the use of restraints. Dr. Fletcher, who had instituted a hospital-wide reform of banning restraints, replied to Mr. Thayer in the *Indianapolis News* that Indiana could not furnish the money to provide skilled and properly educated attendants. Mr. Thayer noticed no difference in the treatment of patients at the hospital between Republican and Democratic administrations of state government. He died in 1914.

## John Zwara[1-4]

Jan [John] Zwara was born in Horni Stepanov, Hungary on December 27, 1880. His parents, Joseph and Mary Zwara, eventually moved the family to Turdossin, Slovakia. He received a primary and high school education and then spent one year at the Academy of Fine Art in Prague, Czechoslovakia and then three more years at the Warsaw Academy of Art in Poland.

At the urging of his brother, Zwara came to Chicago in 1902 at age twenty-two. His brother set him up in an art studio, but John suffered the onset of schizophrenia and began wandering around the United States. He traveled to many states including Ohio, Pennsylvania, Wisconsin, Montana, Nevada, California, Colorado, and Utah, moving from job to job working in mines, smelters, ranches, lumber camps, and on the railroad. His longest job was working for six years on the Los Angeles aqueduct. While taking menial jobs, he nursed his talents as a painter of landscapes and flowers.

Zwara finally settled in Omaha, Nebraska in about 1922 and stayed there for nine years before coming to Indianapolis around 1933. While living in Omaha he became a successful painter and sold many of his paintings to avid art collectors who appreciated his considerable artistic talents. While in Omaha, Zwara carried around a manuscript, partly written in English and partly in other languages. It contained mathematical and other symbols, bits and pieces of philosophy, and Zwara would not let it get out of his sight. Once he threw some of his pictures off the Douglas Street Bridge in Omaha.

After arriving in Indianapolis, Kurt Lieber's art supply company sold Zwara art supplies, paid him one dollar per painting and sold them for five dollars. Then around 1934, Alexander Vonnegut, uncle to author Kurt Vonnegut, Jr. and an admirer of Zwara's paintings, befriended Zwara and even invited him to the family's lake cottage on Lake Maxinkuckee in northern Indiana. By that time Zwara was neglecting his personal hygiene and Vonnegut's wife would not have him in the house so he slept in the barn.

In about 1938 Vonnegut arranged for Zwara's commitment and admission to Central State Hospital. On the admission papers, Vonnegut reported, "Since I have known the patient he has been mighty queer; incapable of handling money...[he] can give an account of himself only incoherently. He is perfectly articulate with paint and paper...Zwara has slept under bridges and in public parks...he is hopelessly disoriented." Dr. Murray DeArmond was one of the two psychiatrists who opined that Mr. Zwara was insane. On admission he was described as rambling, incoherent, and delusional. Dr. Walter Bruetsch diagnosed Zwara as suffering from dementia praecox or schizophrenia. While Zwara was at Central State Hospital he was supplied with art supplies with which he painted scenes of the hospital grounds, including the pathology building, greenhouse, gardens, the distant Indianapolis skyline, and the seven steeples women's building. Zwara left Central State after about six months to resume his peripatetic lifestyle. He made numerous trips to Brown County, Indiana to paint scenes there. He also painted the Butler University campus and scenes from White River. His paintings were exhibited by the Hoosier Salon in 1937, 1943, 1944, and 1945.

After leaving Central State Hospital Zwara continued to live in the Indianapolis area and was eventually taken in by the Little Sisters of the Poor. He died of a cerebral hemorrhage on May 4, 1951.

# Afterword

"Those who cannot remember the past are condemned to repeat it."

George Santayana,
*Reason in Common Sense*, 1905

In Indiana's beginnings, first as a territory and then as a state, the mentally ill were kept in poor houses and jails. Over the past two decades a disturbing trend has surfaced both in Indiana and many other states; as mental state mental hospitals have been downsized or outright closed, the mentally ill population in our nation's jails has skyrocketed. In Indiana Beatty Memorial Hospital has been converted into the Westville Correctional Facility and the New Castle State Developmental Center has been converted into the New Castle Correctional Facility while Madison State Hospital has given up a majority of its real estate to the Madison Correctional Facility [for women].

In 1998 Lamb and Weinberger published an article in *Psychiatric Services* mentioning that studies show that ten to fifteen percent of prisoners in jails and prisons are severely mentally ill and are receiving psychotropic medication.[1] Since their definition of severe mental illness did not include alcohol or substance abuse, the proportion of mentally ill in our jails and prisons skyrockets far beyond fifteen percent.

E. Fully Torrey has characterized our jails and prisons as being "America's new mental hospitals." He indicated that the Los Angeles County jail system, of whose twenty-one thousand inmates thirty-three hundred were severely mentally ill, had become the "largest mental institution in the country."[2]

193

Torrey's most recent study is downright shocking.[3] He found that in 2004-05 there were three times more seriously mentally ill individuals in the United States correctional system than in psychiatric hospital beds. From 1983 to 2009 the percentage of seriously mentally ill persons in jails and prisons has jumped from six percent to seventeen percent. This increase is inversely proportional to the decline in psychiatric beds in general and psychiatric hospitals. For example, in 1955 there was one psychiatric bed for every three hundred persons in the United States, but in 2005 there was only one bed for every three thousand persons. Looking at the problem in a slightly different way, about forty percent of persons with serious mental illnesses have been incarcerated at some point in their lives.

Where is Indiana compared to the other states? Indiana ranks twenty-seventh in expenditures by state mental health authorities. Indiana has an estimated number of 6,393 seriously mentally ill persons incarcerated and 2,413 persons occupying a psychiatric bed. Thus, we have 2.6 times more seriously mentally ill persons in jails and prisons that in psychiatric beds. Indiana followed the lead of other states in closing state hospitals, not heeding outcome data from those states that indicated only moderate success in integrating most seriously mentally ill persons into community living.

Unfortunately the treatment offered to mentally ill prisoners does not begin to compare with that offered in a modern mental hospital setting. In my [Coons] work as a forensic psychiatrist over the past twenty years I have observed this firsthand. At one county jail I encountered a mentally ill prisoner who was getting neither medication for his psychosis nor medication for his acquired immunodeficiency syndrome. At a large new Indiana Department of Corrections facility, ostensibly built to house mentally ill offenders, a psychotic prisoner who had stripped off all of his clothing was thought by correctional staff to be faking. Although efforts to correct these problems have been initiated, these represent a drop in the bucket.[4]

Lamb and Weinberger made a number of suggestions to reverse the disturbing trend described above. They suggest mental health training of police and correctional officers, mental health screening of all incoming inmates, diversion of mentally ill defendants into treatment programs, and the use of more assertive case treatment and outpatient commitments to prevent incarceration.

But do Lamb and Weinberger's suggestions go far enough? Our legislators have de facto decided that it is cheaper to treat the mentally ill in prison rather that in mental hospitals and they have increasingly criminalized mental illness, especially drug and alcohol abuse. Strict rules have limited prison formularies so that mentally ill offenders do not benefit from many of the newer psychotropic medications. In many states treatment consists mainly of medication. Most correctional officers are not trained in dealing with mentally ill offenders. Our prisons' supermax facilities actually worsen mental illness via sensory deprivation in isolation cells. When offenders are released on probation, they often cannot afford to pay for probation services so their probations are revoked and they are re-incarcerated. Even when ex-offenders are released after probation, they often re-offend because they cannot find employment and are sent back to prison. We would suggest that the total cost to society from incarcerating the mentally ill is far beyond a simple comparison between what it costs to hospitalize an individual and what it costs to imprison that same person. We would also suggest that our legislators reverse this trend towards the criminalization of mental illness by providing not only more diversion programs but by increasing state mental hospital beds, relaxing penalties for drug possession, and legislating treatment before incarceration.

It is hard to be optimistic. As we write this, our nation is just emerging from a severe recession. Tax revenues in Indiana have plummeted and Governor Mitchell Daniels has just announced the second series of across-the-board cuts to state agency budgets. In the latest cut there will be a net closure of 355 state psychiatric hospital beds, representing a thirty percent decrease in current capacity. The remaining mental retardation/developmental disability beds in our state hospitals are to be phased out and inpatient youth service and alcohol/substance abuse programs are being closed at Richmond State Hospital. Although the number of forensic beds for serious mental illness are being increased, there is a net loss of inpatient beds for civil patients with serious mental illnesses.[5] It is unclear what the new national healthcare reform law and new mental health treatment parity laws will have on the nation's mental health system.

Crisis always brings an opportunity for change, however, so there is room for optimism in public mental health. We hold even greater optimism for the future of psychiatric treatment as knowledge is burgeoning about the basis of mental illness, enabling the development of more effective psychotherapies and medications for treatment. As treatment for mental illness progresses in the twenty-first century, we call for our state's mental health systems to reverse their current trend towards a return to the nineteenth century practice of treatment in jails and prisons.

# Chapter Notes and References

## Introduction

1. Kennedy, Sheila. The poor you have always with you. In David Bodenhamer and Randall Shepard (Eds.), *The History of Indiana Law*. Athens, Ohio: Ohio University Press, 2006, pp. 90-109.
2. Dix, Dorothea. Jails and poor houses in Indiana. *Indiana State Journal* [Indianapolis]. August 17, 1847 to October 19, 1847.
3. Dix, Dorothea. *Indiana State Journal* [Indianapolis], August 17, 1847.
4. Dix, Dorothea. *Indiana State Journal* [Indianapolis], August 24, 1847.
5. Dix, Dorothea. *Indiana State Journal* [Indianapolis], September 7, 1847.
6. Dix, Dorothea. *Indiana State Journal* [Indianapolis], September 21, 1847.
7. Dix, Dorothea. *Indiana State Journal* [Indianapolis], September 28, 1847.
8. Dix, Dorothea. *Indiana State Journal* [Indianapolis], October 11, 1847.
9. Dix, Dorothea. *Indiana State Journal* [Indianapolis], October 19, 1847

## Chapter 1 A brief history of psychiatry in the United States

1.  Rush, Benjamin. *Medical Inquiries and Observations upon the Diseases of the Mind.* Philadelphia, Pennsylvania: Kimber and Richardson, 1812.

2.  Van Atta, Kim, Roby, David S., and Roby, R. Ross. An account of the events surrounding the origin of Friends Hospital & a brief description of the early years of Friends Asylum, 1817-1820. Philadelphia, Pennsylvania: Friends Hospital, 1980.

3.  American Psychiatric Association. *Diagnostic and Statistical Manual of Mental Disorders.* Washington DC: American Psychiatric Association, 1952.

4.  Ray, Isaac. *A Treatise on the Medical Jurisprudence of Insanity.* Boston, 1838.

5.  Colp, Ralph. History of psychiatry. In Benjamin Sadock &Virginia Sadock (Eds.), *Kaplan and Sadock's comprehensive textbook of psychiatry* (Vol. 2, seventh edition). Philadelphia, Pennsylvania: Lippincott Williams & Wilkins, 2000, pp. 3301-3332.

6.  Harmon, Rebecca B. 2009. Hydrotherapy in state mental hospitals in the mid-twentieth century. *Issues in Mental Health Nursing,* 30:491-494.

7.  [Nursing] *Student manual.* Logansport, Indiana: Logansport State Hospital, 1957.

8.  Goodman, Barak, and Maggio, John. American Experience: The lobotomist. Public Broadcasting Service. http://www.pbs. org/wgbh/americanexperience/films/lobotomist/

9.  Forrer, Gordon, and Miller, Jacob. 1958. Atropine coma: A somatic therapy in psychiatry, *American Journal of Psychiatry,* 115: 455-458.

10. Gazdag, Gábor, Bitter, István, Ungvári, Gábor, and Gerevich, Josef. 2005. Atropine coma: A historical note. *Journal of ECT,* 21:203-206.

11. Levy, David. 1952. Critical evaluation of the present state of child psychiatry. *American Journal of Psychiatry,* 108:481-494.

12. Dwyer, Ellen. *Homes for the mad: Life inside two nineteenth-century asylums.* New Brunswick: Rutgers University Press, 1987.

## Chapter 2 Central State Hospital (1848-1994): Indiana's First Public Psychiatric Hospital

1. *Mental hygiene in Indiana.* Indianapolis, Indiana: State of Indiana Department of Public Welfare, 1950.
2. Family & Social Services Administration, Division of Mental Health and Addictions. Admission/Discharge/Enrollment Summary. http://www.in.gov/fssa/dmha/4672.htm
3. Maisel, Albert. Bedlam1946: Most US mental hospitals are a shame and a disgrace. *Life Magazine*, May 6, 1946, pp. 100-118.
4. Maisel, Albert. Scandal results in real reform: Aroused by the expose of five years ago, state are bringing mental hospitals – and inmates – back from bedlam. *Life Magazine*, November 12, 1951, pp. 140-148.

### Hospital Construction

1. Thomas S. Kirkbride. *On the construction, organization, and general arrangements of hospitals for the insane with some remarks on insanity and its treatment* (2nd edition). Philadelphia, Pennsylvania: J.P. Lippincott, 1880.

### Central State Hospital

1. Bahr, Max. Centennial Anniversary of Central State Hospital Indianapolis, Indiana. Sunday, Nov. 21, 1948.
2. Williams, Clifford L. *A history of mental hospitals in Indiana.* Indianapolis, Indiana, 1960.
3. Hurd, Henry M., Drewry, William F., Dewey, Richard, et al. *The institutional care of the insane in the United States and Canada*, Vol. 2. Baltimore, Maryland: Johns Hopkins Press, 1916, pp. 322-338.
4. Hazelrigg, Charles. 1981. Central State Hospital. *Indiana Medical History Quarterly*, 7(3):3-11.
5. Care of the insane still top state problem. *Indianapolis Star*, September 27, 1953.
6. Miler, Dennis. Asylum. *Indiana State Board of Health Bulletin.* May, 1975, 3-4.

7.  Karsell, Thomas G. Ancient Central State Hospital has space-age ideas on care. *Indianapolis Star*, April 11, 1964.

8.  The Central Hospital for the Insane, situated west of the city has as large population as an ordinary county seat town. *Indianapolis Star*, May 15, 1904.

9.  Cavinder, Fred D. Renewed doses of old medicine. *Indianapolis Star Magazine*, July 30, 1978.

10. McDonnell, Katherine M. 1987. The old pathology building: The Indiana Medical History Museum's most priceless artifact. *Indiana Medicine*, 80:1190-1194.

11. Bahr, Max A. 1931. Mending crippled minds with modern therapeutic aids. *Modern Hospital*, 37(6):1-5.

12. Hendrie, Hugh C. 1983. Press coverage of Central State Hospital: Alarms and excursions. *Indiana Medical History Quarterly*, 11: 5-12.

13. Dwyer, Ellen. 1983. Mental health care in the early twentieth century Indiana and the limits of reform. *Indiana Medical History Quarterly*, 9: 23-27.

14. Central State Hospital discharge study. Indiana University Institute for Social Research.

15. Dean, Eric T. *Shook over hell: Post-traumatic stress, Vietnam, and the Civil War.* Cambridge, Massachusetts: Harvard University Press, 1997.

16. McDougal, Robert A. *The Central State Hospital cemetery list.* Indianapolis, Indiana: Genealogical Society of Marion County, 2000.

## Chapter 3 Public Psychiatric Hospitals Built in the Late Nineteenth Century

### Logansport State Hospital

1.  History of Logansport State Hospital. Logansport, Indiana: Logansport State Hospital, 1956.

2.  A brief history of Logansport State Hospital. 1963. *Indiana History Bulletin*, 40(6): 87-91.

3.  *Superintendent's Report: Thirty-eighth year of the Northern Indiana Hospital for the Insane for the fiscal year ending September 30, 1926.* Indianapolis, Indiana: William B. Burford,1927.

4. Preparation for Longcliff took five years. *Pharos Tribune and Logansport Press*, July 21, 1963.

5. Logansport State Hospital Community Relations Committee. *Logansport State Hospital.* Logansport Indiana: Logansport State Hospital Community Relations Committee.

6. Longcliff plagued with personnel problems. *Pharos Tribune and Logansport Press*, July 21, 1963.

7. Nursing service largest Longcliff department. *Pharos Tribune and Logansport Press*, July 21, 1963.

8. Maisel, Albert. Scandal results in real reform: Aroused by the expose of five years ago, state are bringing mental hospitals – and inmates – back from bedlam. *Life Magazine*, November 12, 1951, pp. 140-148.

9. Social service program department started at state hospital in 1941. *Pharos Tribune and Logansport Press*, July 21, 1963.

10. Musical therapy in Logansport Hospital has important place in patients' treatment. *Indianapolis Star*, May 25, 1952.

11. Smallpox caused Longcliff crisis. *Pharos Tribune and Logansport Press*, July 21, 1963.

12. Water has been a big problem at hospital. *Pharos Tribune and Logansport Press*, July 21, 1963.

13. Temperature again climbs past 100 mark. *Logansport Pharos Tribune*, July 27, 1936.

14. Blame heat for death of patient. *Logansport Pharos Tribune*, July 28, 1936.

15. Longcliff fire threat kept to a minimum. *Pharos Tribune and Logansport Press*, July 21, 1963.

16. Longcliff grounds now cover over 1300 acres. *Pharos Tribune and Logansport Press*, July 21, 1963.

17. Logansport State Hospital dairy…a while ago. 2007. *Spectrum.* Logansport, Indiana: Logansport State Hospital, 17(6): 7-8.

18. Logansport State Hospital. *The Logansport State Hospital dedication exercises for the building program.* Logansport, Indiana: Logansport State Hospital, May 13, 1940.

19. *Logansport Pharos Tribune.* February 28, 1951.

20. Hetherington, John, Smith, E. Rogers, Larson, John A., and Ferguson, John. Psychosurgery in the Logansport State Hospital. 1954. *Journal of the Indiana State Medical Association*, 47:1097-1100.

21. Kitchell, Dave. The first 100 years of Longcliff. *Pharos Tribune and Logansport Press*, July 21, 1963.
22. Logansport State Hospital facility fact sheet SFY 2009.
23. Freehafer, Don. Found, companion and friend. *Indianapolis Star Magazine*, November 4, 1960, pp. 7-9, 12.
24. Logansport State Hospital. *Logansport State Hospital Information Handbook*. Logansport, Indiana: Logansport State Hospital.
25. Logansport State Hospital. *Longcliff Museum*. Logansport, Indiana: Logansport State Hospital.
26. Saine, Deb. Longcliff, then and now. *Logansport Pharos Tribune*, June 4, 2000.
27. Brooks, Ralph L. Paint and relax: You might save yourself from a breakdown, for art is well recognized by psychiatrists for its therapeutic value. *Indianapolis Star Magazine*, September 18, 1955, pp. 7-8.
28. Cass County Indiana GenWeb. Cemeteries in Cass County Indiana: Logansport State Hospital Cemetery. http://incass-inmiami.org/cass/cemeteries/abnd/Longcliff/LSHal.html

## Richmond State Hospital

1.  Richmond State Hospital. *Richmond State Hospital remembers 90 years serving east central Indiana*. Richmond, Indiana: Richmond State Hospital,1980.
2.  Land, Dale O. and Harris, Elaine (Eds.). 1990. *100 years at Richmond State Hospital*. Richmond, Indiana: Richmond State Hospital.
3.  Division of Mental Health and Addictions, Family and Social Services Administration. History of Richmond State Hospital. http://www.in.gov/fssa/dmha/2614.htm
4.  Colony for insane to be establish, governor authorizes expenditure of $75,000 for the purchase of land. Site already obtained. Farm will be near Richmond, in Wayne County – preliminary arrangements made by Dr. Smith. *Indianapolis Star*, October 15, 1912.
5.  One dead, another missing in flames at Easthaven. Fire gutted men's hospital ward. *Richmond Palladium Item*, March 6, 1919.

6. Richmond State Hospital Pioneers with shock treatment. *Public Welfare in Indiana*, November, 1938, pp. 6-7.
7. McCord, Al G. Alarm cue for speedy fund action. Hospital shocks [Governor] Craig. *Indianapolis Star*, July 2, 1953.
8. Richmond Hospital in fairly good shape. *Indianapolis Times*, December 7, 1963.
9. Richmond State Hospital. *Annual Report of July 1, 1953 to June 30, 1954*. Richmond Indiana: Richmond State Hospital.
10. Richmond State Hospital. *Annual Report of July 1, 1954 to June 30, 1955*. Richmond Indiana: Richmond State Hospital.
11. Richmond State Hospital. Bill of fare, May 21 to May 27, 1933. Richmond, Indiana: Richmond State Hospital.
12. Richmond State Hospital. Bill of fare, February 9 to February 15, 1936. Richmond, Indiana: Richmond State Hospital.
13. Richmond State Hospital Facility Fact Sheet SFY 2009.

## Evansville State Hospital

1. Evansville State Hospital. *Hospital history*. Evansville, Indiana: Evansville State Hospital.
2. Sampson, Evaline. *History of Woodmere*, about 1945.
3. Lehman, Bill. *Evansville State Hospital: 1890-1990*. Evansville, Indiana: University of Southern, Indiana, August, 1990.
4. The new insane hospital. Something of the new building now being occupied. The official quarters and how patient wards are furnished – yesterday arrivals from Indianapolis. *Evansville Journal*, November 26, 1890.
5. The insane asylum. To be opened for patients on Thursday next. *Evansville Journal*, October 26, 1890
6. Coons, Philip M. 2008. History of psychiatry in Indiana: Evansville State Hospital Fire. *Spectrum* [Indiana Psychiatric Society], 44(4):3.
7. Patients sent to hospitals in other cities. *Evansville Press*, February 10, 1943.
8. To use same hospital site. *Evansville Press*, February 12, 1943.
9. $2,000,000 building to replace burned asylum at Evansville. *Indianapolis Times*, June 25, 1943.

10. Superintendent of Evansville State Hospital fired. *Indianapolis News*, November 15, 1968.
11. 5 doctors quit over Evansville State firing. *Indianapolis Star*, January 16, 1969.
12. Lack of stigma makes operation of Evansville hospital easier. *Indianapolis Star*, April 19, 1964.
13. Evansville State Hospital. *Evansville State Hospital 74-75 annual report*. Evansville, Indiana: Evansville State Hospital, 1975.
14. Evansville State Hospital facility fact sheet SFY 2009.
15. Turner, Sally. Remains will be moved to cemetery. *Evansville Press*, June 23, 1987.

## Chapter 4 Twentieth Century Public Psychiatric Hospitals in Indiana

### Madison State Hospital

1. Revision of an article by Coons, Philip. 2010. Madison State Hospital: Indiana Psychiatry's best kept secret. *Spectrum* (Indiana Psychiatric Society), 44(7):4-5.
2. Zirkle, George (Ed.). Madison State Hospital: The first half century. Madison, Indiana: Madison State Hospital.
3. Eagle, Wayne. MSH museum offers insight into history of mental health care. *Madison Courier*, August 30, 2001.
4. Madison State Hospital. *New employee handbook*. Madison , Indiana: Madison State Hospital.
5. World Architectural News. WorldArchitectureNews. com http://www.worldarchitecturenews.com/index. php?fuseaction=wanappln.projectview&upload_id=921
6. Madison State Hospital. 2007. *The MSH Bulletin*, 10(38):1.
7. Madison State Hospital. Facility fact sheet, SFY 2009.

### Larue D. Carter Memorial Hospital

1. Indiana General Assembly. An act concerning mental cases, creating the Indiana Council for Mental Health and prescribing its powers and duties, authorizing the construction of a hospital, providing for admission thereto and release

therefrom and making an appropriation, and providing for enforcement. *Laws of the state of Indiana, Regular session of the 84th Indiana General Assembly.* Indianapolis, Indiana: Bookwalter Company, 1945, pp. 1571.

2. Larue D. Carter Memorial Hospital. *Larue D. Carter Memorial Hospital, 50 years of serving mental health in Indiana.* Indianapolis, Indiana: Larue D. Carter Memorial Hospital, 2002.

3. Governor breaks ground for new mental hospital. *Indianapolis Star*, January 15, 1948.

4. Budget cut may delay new hospital. *Indianapolis News*, January 22, 1951.

5. Larue D. Carter Hospital to serve state's mentally ill. 1952. *Journal of the Indiana State Medical Association*, 45:1167-1168.

6. Juul C. Nielsen. Another milestone. 1952. *Monthly Bulletin of the Indiana State Board of Health*, 45:195, 213-215.

7. Juul C. Nielsen. Indiana's new approach to mental illness. 1954. Modern Hospital, 82(3):73-77.

8. Larue D. Carter Memorial Hospital. *The Larue D. Carter Memorial Hospital dedication program.* Indianapolis, Indiana: Larue D. Carter Memorial Hospital, September 28, 1952.

9. Recruitment of hospital staff begins. *Indianapolis Star*, December 14, 1951.

10. New hospital but where are doctors? *Indianapolis News*, July 17, 1952.

11. Mental cases rouse mayor: Hits Carter Hospital for not helping out. *Indianapolis Star*, November 14, 1952.

12. Power, Freemont. $5 million hospital half-used, lacks staff: Mentally ill stay in jail. *Indianapolis News*, June 13, 1953.

13. City may lease wing of hospital. *Indianapolis News*, July 23, 1953.

14. Averitt, Jack. Mental hospital to open new space. *Indianapolis Star*, August 8, 1953.

15. Carter Hospital opens new unit for children. *Indianapolis Star*, October 14, 1954.

16. Wilson, John V. Psychiatry spotlights problem boys. *Indianapolis Times*, March 20, 1955.

17. Larue D. Carter Memorial Hospital. *Second annual report of the superintendent of the Larue D. Carter Memorial Hospital at Indianapolis, Indiana for the fiscal year ending June 30, 1954.* Indianapolis, Indiana: Larue D. Carter Memorial Hospital.

18. Wilson, John V. Exodus of psychiatrists cuts treatment of the mentally ill: Official concedes inadequacies at Larue Carter. *Indianapolis Times*, September 11, 1955.

19. Cavinder, Fred D. Minds recalmed. *Indianapolis Star Magazine*, August 5, 1956, pp. 6-8.

20. Child's mental illness causes puzzle psychiatric workers. *Indianapolis Star*, February 23, 1958.

21. Pulliam, Myra. Unlocking of ward doors changes hospitals other ways. *Indianapolis Star*, January 9, 1972.

22. Holmes, Leila. Ex-Larue Carter patients now get evaluation. *Indianapolis Star*, August 18, 1974.

23. Martin, P.J., Moore, J.E., Sterne, A.L., and McNairy, R.M. 1977. Therapists' prophesy. *Journal of Clinical Psychology*, 33:502-510.

24. Larue D. Carter Memorial Hospital. *Larue D. Carter Memorial Hospital* (2nd ed.). Indianapolis, Indiana: Larue D. Carter Memorial Hospital, 1981.

25. Pratt, James and Small, Iver F. *Larue D. Carter Memorial Hospital: A state-wide program for the treatment of resistant patients.* Indianapolis, Indiana: Larue D. Carter Memorial Hospital, 1983.

## Chapter 5 Private Psychiatric Institutions

### Neuronhurst

1. Coons, Philip M. 2005. Drs. William Baldwin Fletcher and Mary Angela Spink: Neuropsychiatrists and Superintendents of Neuronhurst. *Spectrum*, [Indiana Psychiatric Society], 42(2): 5, 9.

2. Neuronhurst is well-known sanitorium. *Indianapolis News*, September 18, 1926.

3. 1930 United States Census Center Township, Marion County, Indiana, E.D. No. 49,

4. S.D. No. 8, sheet 7A, p. 44. 4. Esarey, Logan. *History of Indiana from its exploration to 1922 with an account of Indianapolis and Marion County*, Vol. 4. Dayton, Ohio: Dayton Historical Publishing Company, 1924.

## Norways

1. Coons, Philip M. Early psychiatry in Indiana: Norways Hospital. 2008. *Spectrum* [Indiana Psychiatric Society], 44 (3):1, 7, 10.
2. Reed, Philip B. The private psychiatric hospital. *Psychiatric Services*, 9(2); 34-35.
3. Reed, Philip B. Troubled people.1952. *Monthly Bulletin of the Indiana State Board of Health*, 45(9):200-218.
4. Mickels, Donna. Small local hospital blazed trail in psychiatric medicine. *Indianapolis Times*, June 26, 1949.
5. A dream approaches reality. *Norways Quarterly*, 1952.
6. Sterne, Albert E. 1904. Neurasthenia and its treatment by actinic rays. *Journal of the American Medical Association*, 42:500-507.
7. Norways Hospital. Dr. Robert Bill joins Norways as director of psychotherapy. *Norways Quarterly*, 1956.
8. Norways gets third of grant. *Indianapolis Star*, May 10, 1956.
9. State Ford grants total half million. *Indianapolis Times*, January 18, 1959.
10. New mental hospital will be built here. *Indianapolis Times*, November 20, 1953.
11. Norways Hospital. New Norways will adjoin Methodist. *Norways Quarterly*, 1955.
12. Plan to close Norways bared. *Indianapolis Star*, February 12, 1957.
13. Norways Hospital sets move to smaller city. *Indianapolis Times*, March 31, 1957.
14. Norways' patients to transfer. *Indianapolis Star*, September 22, 1957.
15. Norways' medical chief to take Lafayette post. *Indianapolis News*, September 23, 1957.

## Methodist Hospital

1. Leary, Edward A. 1984. *The history of Methodist Hospital of Indiana, Inc.: A mission of compassionate health care.* Indianapolis, Indiana: Methodist Health Foundation.
2. Williams, Judy. Methodist psychiatric wing ready. *Indianapolis News*, June 11, 1959.
3. Methodist Hospital adds 41-bed psychiatric unit. *Indianapolis News*, June 28, 1968.

## Chapter 6 Developmental Centers

1. Conroy, James W. and Seiders, Jeffrey X. Outcomes of community placement at six months for the people who moved from New Castle and Northern Indiana State Developmental Centers. Report number 4 of the Indiana community placement quality tracking project. September, 1999.
2. West, Evan. Jimmy Sullivan: Two boys. *Indianapolis Monthly*, Vol. 29, December, 2005, pp. 121-125 and 192-196.

### Fort Wayne Developmental Center

1. Thompson, Pamela M. (editor). 2007. *Fort Wayne State Developmental Center, 1879-2007.* Bala Cynwyd, Pennsylvania: Liberty Healthcare.
2. Schwin, Lulu B. Fort Wayne State School. September. 1938. Clipping file, Indiana State Library, Indianapolis, Indiana.
3. Fort Wayne State School. *74th Annual Report of the Fort Wayne State School*, June 30, 1952. Richmond, Indiana: Fort Wayne State School.
4. Model training school being designed for Fort Wayne. *Indianapolis Times*, June 17, 1956.
5. Bloem, Robert. Improvement pledged at "neglected" Fort Wayne institution. Feeble-minded school inspected by new mental health chief. Overcrowded, understaffed home promised aid, but Dr. Zeller says solution is not easy. *Indianapolis Times*, September 25, 1947.
6. Smith, Richhard P. State School, in 68th year, on threshold of better era. *Fort Wayne News Sentinel*, March, 1958.

## New Castle State Developmental Center

1.  New Castle State Hospital. *Valley News.* New Castle: New Castle State Hospital, Vol. 6 (1), July 1980.
2.  Kellum, Robert W. State Village for Epileptics monument to humane spirit. *Indianapolis Star,* June 2, 1946.
3.  New Castle State Village grows its own food; Patients eat well. *Indianapolis Star,* October 17, 1945.
4.  [Indiana Village for Epileptics]. *Indianapolis Star,* June 21, 1925.
5.  Zile, Frankl. Making the way for new look: DOC moves land, demolishes most buildings, construction to begin in a couple of months. *New Castle Courier Times,* August 2, 1999.

## Muscatatuck State Developmental Center

1.  Muscatatuck State Hospital and Training Center. *Annual Report of the Muscatatuck State Hospital and Training Center, 1974.* Butlerville, Indiana: Muscatatuck State Hospital and Training Center.
2.  Deiber, Camilla. Streamlined styles define Muscatatuck. *Indiana Preservationist,* January/February, 1997, pp. 8-9.
3.  Fifer, Orien W. Indiana augments its care of feeble-minded with enlarged village at Muscatatuck. *Indianapolis News,* May 18, 1940.
4.  Red infiltration at Muscatatuck charged; investigation urged. *Indianapolis Times,* May 24, 1957.
5.  West, Evan. Jimmy Sullivan: Two boys. *Indianapolis Monthly,* Vol. 29, December, 2005, pp. 121-125 and 192-196.
6.  Crosby, John. Muscatatuck open house gives locals view of premier Army training site. Muscatatuck Urban Training Center.http://www.mutc.in.ng.mil/

## Northern Indiana State Developmental Center

1.  State offered hospital land. *Indianapolis Star,* August 6, 1946.
2.  Early, Maurice. The day in Indiana. *Indianapolis Star,* July 7, 1950.

## Silvercrest Children's Developmental Center

1. New T.B. Hospital door open today. Silvercrest, New Albany, to provide beds for 150 patients. *Indianapolis Star*, August 1, 1940.
2. Silvercrest: An architectural treasure in the hills of New Albany. New Albany Preservation. http://www.newalbanypreservation. com/uploads/File/Silvercrest%20Site/Silvercrest_History.pdf
3. Silvercrest marks 25 years. *Louisville Courier Journal*, September 4, 1999.
4. Campbell, Eric S. Silvercrest, in New Albany, to house seniors. *Evening News and Tribune*, September 2, 2007.

## Chapter 7 Correctional Facilities

### Indiana State Prison

1. Griffo, Charles G.. Beatty Hospital soon to provide new hope for criminally insane. *Indianapolis Star*, December 21, 1953.

### Norman Beatty Hospital

1. Underwood, Don. State selects site for insane hospital. $136,660 is paid for location on edge of Westville. *Indianapolis News*, June 5, 1946.
2. Beatty Hospital erases need to jail mentally ill. *Indianapolis Star*, January 30, 1952.
3. New mental hospital to be complete city. *Indianapolis News*, July 21, 1949.
4. Griffo, Charles G. Beatty Hospital marks new mental health era. *Indianapolis Star*, July 27, 1952.
5. Griffo, Charles G. New mental hospital is a city unto itself. *Indianapolis Star*, January 28, 1952.
6. Beatty Hospital erases need to jail mentally ill. *Indianapolis Star*, January 30, 1952.
7. Griffo, Charles G. Beatty Hospital soon to provide new hope for criminally insane. *Indianapolis Star*, December 21, 1953.
8. Griffo, Charles G. Help poses problem for Beatty Hospital. *Indianapolis Star*, January 29, 1952.

9. Beatty can't become prison, says doctor. *Indianapolis News,* September 29, 1956.

10. Beatty Hospital chief resigns. *Indianapolis News,* December 20, 1967.

11. Thomas, Jason. Despite 2,000 open beds, state outsources inmates; The use of a Kentucky prison to save money turns into a hot topic in the governor's race. *Indianapolis Star,* October 29, 2004.

## Chapter 8 Community Mental Health Centers

1. Stephens, Joseph D. Brief history of the community mental health centers in Indiana. Lawrenceburg, Indiana: Community Mental Health Center, Inc. http://www.iccmhc.org/files/History%20of%20Community%20Mental%20Health%20in%20Indiana.pdf

2. Indiana General Assembly. An act authorizing counties to furnish financial assistance for constructing and operating community mental health centers and community mental retardation centers. *Laws of the state of Indiana passed at the ninety fourth regular session of the General Assembly.* Indianapolis, Indiana: Central Publishing Company, 1965, pp. 78-79.

3. Mental health center to open. *Indianapolis News,* November 3, 1969.

4. Gallahue Center a leader in mental health care. *Indianapolis Star,* January 1, 1976.

## Chapter 9 Psychiatric Organizations

### Division of Mental Health and Addictions

1. Indiana General Assembly. An act concerning mental cases, creating the Indiana Council for Mental Health and prescribing its powers and duties, authorizing the construction of a hospital, providing for admission thereto and release therefrom and making an appropriation, and providing for enforcement. *Laws of the state of Indiana passed at the ninety-second regular session of the Indiana General Assembly.* Indianapolis, Indiana: Bookwalter Company, 1945, pp. 1569-1570.

2.  Indiana General Assembly. An act concerning mental health; providing for the abolition of the Division of Mental Health of the Department of Health and the transfer of rights, powers, duties, functions, authority, and appropriations of the Division of Mental Health of the Department of Health to the Department of Mental Health; creating a division of Child Mental Health in the Department of Mental Health; creating a Division of Mental Retardation in the Department of Mental Health; making an appropriation; and repealing all laws in conflict therewith. *Laws of the state of Indiana, Regular session of the 84th Indiana General Assembly.* Indianapolis, Indiana: Bookwalter Company, 1961, pp. 107-125.

3.  Indiana Council for Mental Health. *Annual report of the Indiana Council for Mental Health of the State of Indiana.* Indianapolis, Indiana: Indiana Council for Mental Health, June 30, 1946.

4.  George Parker. Personal communication, April 2010.

## Indiana Psychiatric Society

1.  Revision of an article by Bowman, Elizabeth S. The earliest days of organized psychiatry in Indiana. 1986. *Indiana Psychiatric Society Newsletter,* 23(3):1, 3, 7, 10.

2.  Revision of an article by Bowman, Elizabeth S. War and the hospitals: INPA in the 1940s. 1987. *Indiana Psychiatric Society Newsletter,* 24(2): 3, 8.

3.  Revision of an article by Bowman, Elizabeth S. 1987. Getting started again: INPA in the early 50s. *Indiana Psychiatric Society Newsletter,* 24(4): 4, 7, 10.

## Northern Indiana Psychiatric Society

1.  1. Matthew, J.H. Northern Indiana Psychiatric Society. In History of the district branches and of the district branch assembly. American Psychiatric Association. http://www.psych.org/MainMenu/EducationCareerDevelopment/Library/APAHistory/AssemblyDistrictBranchesHistory.aspx

## Indiana Mental Health Association

1. Milk, Harry. *The history of the Mental Health Association in Indiana.* Indianapolis, Indiana: Indiana Mental Health Foundation, 1966.

## Chapter 10 Department of Psychiatry, Indiana University School of Medicine

### Introduction

1. Nurnberger, John I. Sr. History of the department of psychiatry. Indianapolis, Indiana: Department of Psychiatry, Indiana University School of Medicine.
2. Nurnberger, John I. Sr., Hendrie, H.C., et. al. History of the department of psychiatry. Indianapolis, Indiana: Department of Psychiatry, Indiana University School of Medicine.

### Residency Training

1. Residents in psychiatry at Indiana University.
2. *Residency training program.* Indianapolis, Indiana: Indiana University School of Medicine, Department of Psychiatry, 1960.
3. Photo composites of Psychiatry resident staff, Indiana University Medical Center. 1964-1965, 1965-1966, 1967-1968, 1968-1969.

### Section of Psychology

1. Indiana University School of Medicine Psychology Internship Program. Department of Psychiatry, Indiana University School of Medicine. http://psychiatry.medicine.iu.edu/body.cfm?id=62

### Institute of Psychiatric Research

1. State takes $1,000,000 mental research stride. *Indianapolis Star*, December 4, 1956.

2.  Institute of Psychiatric Research. *First annual report of the Institute of Psychiatric Research of the Department of Psychiatry, Indiana University Medical Center, and Division of Mental Health the State of Indiana.* Indianapolis, Indiana: Indiana University School of Medicine, July 1, 1957 to June 30, 1958.

3.  Institute of Psychiatric Research. *Second annual report of the Institute of Psychiatric Research under the Department of Psychiatry, Indiana University Medical Center, and Division of Mental Health, the State of Indiana.* Indianapolis, Indiana: Indiana University School of Medicine, July 1, 1958 to June 30, 1959.

## Long Adult Psychiatry Clinic

1.  Kooiker, John E. and Lubin, Bernard. 1962. The adult psychiatry clinic at Indiana University Medical Center: Services and patient population. *Journal of the Indiana State Medical Association,* 8:1158- 1161.

## Marion County General Hospital

1.  To treat the deranged: Detention department will be established at City Hospital. *Indianapolis News,* April 9, 1907.

## Chapter 11 Child psychiatry

1.  Kanner, Leo. *Child Psychiatry.* London: Balliere, Tindall, and Cox, 1935.

## Early Child Guidance Clinics at Indiana University School of Medicine

1.  Undated and untitled manuscript, probably written in 1959.

## Riley Child Psychiatry Clinic

1.  Newell, Robert. Clinics for problem kids pay dividends. *Indianapolis News,* May 31, 1949.
2.  Junior League votes $75,000 for Riley Child Guidance Clinic. *Indianapolis News,* April 22, 1947.

3. Simmons, James E. 1960. Child psychiatry in Indiana. *Journal of the Indiana State Medical Association*, 53:1348-1356.
4. Weinberg, Mary. League center turns problem child into happy one. *Indianapolis News*, December 10, 1949.
5. Riley Clinic head named. *Indianapolis News*, January 1, 1951.
6. Child guidance clinic opens second office. *Indianapolis Star*, January 31, 1978.

## Marion County Child Guidance Clinic

1. Newell, Robert. Scope is outlined. *Indianapolis News*, May 24, 1949.
2. Child guidance clinic to open. *Indianapolis Star*, January 29, 1950.
3. Lewis, Carl. Leaning post for parents. *Indianapolis Star Magazine*, February 19, 1950.
4. Dr. Simmons directs child guidance clinic. *Indianapolis Star*, February 8, 1953.
5. Holmes, Leila. Guidance Clinic director explains role. *Indianapolis Star*, January 30, 1972.

## Evansville Children's Psychiatric Hospital

1. Folz, Edna. Children's psychiatric center explained. *Evansville Press*, February 20, 1964.
2. Evansville Children's Psychiatric Hospital. *Evansville Psychiatric Children's Center: A residential treatment facility for emotionally disturbed children*. Evansville, Indiana: Evansville Children's Psychiatric Hospital.
3. Evansville Children's Psychiatric Hospital. *Evansville Psychiatric Children's Center Annual Report*, 1976-1977. Evansville, Indiana: Evansville Children's Psychiatric Hospital.
4. Native of St. Louis to head child clinic. *Evansville Press*, November 10, 1965.
5. Flynn, Robert. Funds slashed for child center. Evansville Press, March 1, 1969.
6. Bill ok's staffing at children's center. *Evansville Press*, March 27, 1975.

7. Evansville Psychiatric Children's Center. Closing not debatable. "This is starting to stink," says facility's psychiatrist. *Evansville Courier Press*, April 3, 2002.

8. Whitson, Jennifer. Children's center saved at 11th hour. Governor to sign budget bill. *Evansville Courier Press,* June 23, 2002.

## Chapter 12 Notable Indiana Psychiatrists of the Nineteenth Century

### James S. Athon

1. Hazelrigg, Charles. 1981. Central State Hospital. *Indiana Medical History Quarterly*, 7(3):7-8.

2. James S. Athon. In W.W. Wollen (Ed.), *Biographical and historical sketches of early Indiana*, 1883.

### George Frederick Edenharter

1. Dr. G.F. Edenharter to be buried today. Body to lie in state at Central Hospital – Masons plan services. *Indianapolis Star*, December 18, 1923.

2. Dunn, Jacob Pratt. George F. Edenharter, M.D. Greater Indianapolis: The history, the industries, the institutions, and the people of a city of homes. Chicago: Lewis Publishing Company, 1910, pp. 975-978.

3. Early, Maurice. Indiana alienist of national renown through efforts to reduce insanity. Hundreds of physicians will join in celebration Tuesday of Dr. George E. Edenharter's thirtieth anniversary as executive of state hospital – "Live right," is his advice to the public. *Indianapolis Star*, April 29, 1923.

4. George F. Edenharter, M.D. *Pictorial and Biographical Memoirs, Indianapolis and Marion County, Indiana*. Chicago: Goodspeed Brothers Publishers, 1893, pp.35-36.

5. King, Lucy Jane. Indiana's man for all seasons. Speech given at the Indiana Medical History Museum, Indianapolis, Indiana, September 21, 2002. (http://www.morrisswadener.com/notes.html)

## Orpheus Everts

1.  1. American Psychiatric Association. Orpheus Everts, M.D. 1826-1903. American Psychiatric Association. http://www. psychiatry.org/MainMenu/EducationCareerDevelopment/ Library/APAHistory/APA-Presidents-Biographical-Sketches/13-1885-1886-Everts-Orpheus.aspx?css=print
2.  Dr. Everts of Cincinnati [Obituary]. 1910. *Indiana Medical Journal.* 3:76-77.
3.  Hurd, Henry M., Drewry, William F., Dewey, Richard, et al. Dr. Orpheus Everts. *The institutional care of the insane in the United States and Canada*, Vol. 4. Baltimore, Maryland: Johns Hopkins Press, 1917, pp. 394-395.
4.  Orpheus Everts, M.D. [Obituary]. 1903. *Journal of the American Medical Association*, 41:46-47.

## William Baldwin Fletcher

1.  Biographic sketch. Undated and unpublished.
2.  Dr. W.B. Fletcher dies in Florida. *Indianapolis News*, April 25, 1907, p. 1.
3.  Drenovsky, Rachael L. Humanity's bonfire: William B. Fletcher, M.D., 1937-1907. *Traces*, Spring, 2001, pp. 19-25.
4.  Hazelrigg, Charles. 1981. Central State Hospital. *Indiana Medical History Quarterly*, 7(3):3-11.
5.  Indiana Historical Society. Biographical sketch of William Baldwin Fletcher. (Undated manuscript).

## Joseph Goodwin Rogers

1.  American Psychiatric Association. Joseph G. Rogers, M.D. (1841-1908). American Psychiatric Association. http:// psychiatry.org/MainMenu/EducationCareerDevelopment/ Library/APAHistory/APA-Presidents-Biographical-Sketches/27-1899-1900-Rogers-Joseph-G.aspx
2.  Dr. Joseph G. Rogers dead at Logansport. Long the head of the Northern Indiana Hospital for the Insane, eminent as an alienist. *Indianapolis News*, April 4, 1908.
3.  Hessler, Robert. Joseph G. Rogers [Obituary]. 1908. *Journal of the Indiana State Medical Association*, 1:205-206.

4.  Smith, Samuel E. Dr. Joseph Goodwin Rogers. *Sixty-fourth annual meeting of the American Medico-Psychological Association.* Cincinnati, Ohio: American Medico-Psychological Association, May 1908.
5.  Joseph G. Rogers. The state and its insane. *Indiana Bulletin of the Charities and Corrections,* March, 1898, pp. 97-103
6.  Joseph G. Rogers. Presidential Address: A century of hospital building for the insane. *Proceedings of the American Medico-Psychological Association,* Fifty-Sixth Annual Meeting held in Richmond, Virginia, May 22-25, 1900. American Medico-Psychological Association, 1900, pp. 70-87.

## Mary Angela Spink

1.  Dr. Mary Angela Spink, 75, dies, president of Fletcher Sanitarium. *Indianapolis Star,* September 7, 1939
2.  Dunn, Jacob Pratt (Ed.). Mary Angela Spink. *Greater Indianapolis: The history, the industries, the institutions, and the people of a city of homes.* Chicago: Lewis Publishing Company, 1910, vol. 2, pp. 955-956.
3.  Esarey, Logan. *History of Indiana from its exploration to 1922 with an account of Indianapolis and Marion County,* Vol. 4. Dayton, Ohio: Dayton Historical Publishing Company, 1924.

## Albert Eugene Sterne

1.  Brown, Paul (Ed.). Albert E. Sterne. *Indianapolis Men of Affairs.* Indianapolis, Indiana: American Biographical Society, 1923, pp. 582-583.
2.  Dr. Albert E. Sterne dies of heart disease in Denver: Nationally known authority on nervous and mental diseases founded and was chief of Norways Sanitarium – Also professor at I.U. Medical School. *Indianapolis Star,* July 1, 1931.

## Sarah E. Stockton

1.  Dr. Stockton dies after long illness: Widely known woman physician was on staff of Central Hospital for 25 years. *Indianapolis Star,* March 14, 1924.

2. Indiana Commission on Public Records. Sarah E. Stockton (1842-1924). Indiana Commission on Public Records. http://www.in.gov/icpr/2713.htm

3. Sarah Stockton [Obituary]. 1924. *Journal of the Indiana State Medical Association*, 17: 129.

### Andrew J. Thomas

1. Dr. Andrew J. Thomas [Obituary]. 1898. *Indiana Medical Journal*, 17:36

## Chapter 13 Notable Indiana Psychiatrists of the Twentieth Century

1. American Psychiatric Association. *Biographical Directory of the American Psychiatric Association*. Washington, DC: American Psychiatric Association, 1989.

### Clare M. Assue

1. Clara Assue Brown had been medical director at Larue, *Indianapolis Star*, August 30, 1990.

2. Morton, Philip M. Psychiatrist, educator, community leader, Clare M. Assue, M.D., dies. *Indiana Psychiatric Society Newsletter*, October, 1990, pp. 7,9.

3. Sharpley, Patricia, Morton, Philip M., Fisher, William P. Memorial resolution on behalf of Clare M. Assue, M.D., Professor of Psychiatry, Indiana University School of Medicine. Indianapolis, Indiana: Indiana University School of Medicine, September 1991.

### Max A. Bahr

1. Bruetsch, Walter L. In memoriam: Max A. Bahr, M.D., 1874-1953. 1953. *American Journal of Psychiatry*, 109:800.

2. Double honors come in day for Dr. Bahr. *Indianapolis Star*, March 22, 1946.

3. Dr. Bahr, pioneer psychiatrist dies. *Indianapolis News*, June 24, 1953.

4. 500 honor Dr. Bahr, retiring hospital chief. *Indianapolis Star*, January 11, 1952.

5. Max A. Bahr. Biographical sketch, 1935.
6. Tribute to Max A. Bahr, M.D. on the occasion of his retirement as superintendent of Central State Hospital. 1952. *Journal of the Indiana State Medical Association,* 45:314-315.
7. Law students study insanity. *Indianapolis Star,* January 11, 1923.
8. Bahr, Max A. and Bruetsch, Walter A. 1928. Two years' experience with the malarial treatment of general paresis in a state institution: Clinical, serological, and autopsy observation in 100 cases. *American Journal of Psychiatry,* 84:715-727.
9. Bahr, Max A. 1931. Mending crippled minds with modern therapeutic aids. *Modern Hospital,* 37(6):1-6.
10. Bahr, Max A. 1930. Psychiatric problems in children. *Journal of the Indiana State Medical Association,* 23:7-11.
11. Bahr, Max A. My fifty years in psychiatry. Unpublished lecture, January 10, 1952.

### David A. Boyd, Jr.

1. City psychiatric head is named: Dr. David A. Boyd to be full-time hospital director. *Indianapolis Star,* September 24, 1944.
2. I.U. psychiatrist quits to take Mayo Clinic post. *Indianapolis News,* August 9, 1948.
3. Michigan doctor is appointed head of department at I.U. medical unit. *Indianapolis Star,* September 14, 1939.

### Larue Depew Carter

1. Bonsett, Charles. 1977. Larue D. Carter. *Indiana Medical History Quarterly,* 3(2):23-25.
2. Dr. Cater, 65, psychiatrist, lecturer, dies. *Indianapolis Star,* January 22, 1946.
3. Letter dated March 10, 1977 from Philip B. Reed, M.D., to Donald F. Moore, M.D.

### Murray DeArmond

1. Rites for Dr. DeArmond, former psychiatrist, will be Tuesday. *Indianapolis Star,* January 10, 1988.

## Marian Kendall DeMyer

1.  DeMyer, Marian K. *Parents and children in autism.* New York, New York: V.H. Winston, 1979.
2.  Fellows, Ann. Women in the news: Dr. Marian DeMyer. *Indianapolis Times,* August 3, 1961.
3.  William E. DeMyer. [Obituary] Indianapolis Star, September 24, 2008.

## John Thacker Ferguson

1.  De Kruif, Paul. *A man against insanity.* London: Hutchinson & Co., 1958.
2.  Hetherington, John, Smith, E. Rogers, Larson, John A., and Ferguson, John. 1954. Psychosurgery in the Logansport State Hospital. *Journal of the Indiana State Medical Association,* 47:1097-1100.
3.  Logansport State Hospital. *Annual report – 1952-1953.* Logansport, Indiana: Logansport State Hospital.
4.  Logansport State Hospital. *Annual report – 1953-1954.* Logansport, Indiana: Logansport State Hospital.
5.  John Ferguson. [Obituary] *Montreal Gazette,* March 4, 1968.

## William P. Fisher

1.  Bowman, Elizabeth, Landy, Mary and Hendrie, Hugh. Memorial resolution on behalf of William Paul Fisher, M.D., Emeritus Professor of Psychiatry, October 27, 1929 – February 14, 1998. Indianapolis, Indiana: Indiana University School of Medicine, September 3, 1998.
2.  Dr. William Paul Fisher earned honors as psychiatry professor. *Indianapolis Star,* February 18, 1998.

## Ernest J. Fogel

1.  Dr. Fogel named hospital superintendent. *Indianapolis News,* December 12, 1957.
2.  State hospital chief resigns. *Indianapolis News,* August 22, 1967.

3. Superintendent retires. *Indianapolis News*, January 2, 1976.

## Richard N. French

1. Richard N. French. [Obituary] *Indianapolis Star*, January 29, 2005.

## Herbert Stockton Gaskill

1. Dr. Gaskill quits IU post: Will leave position at the medical center. *Indianapolis Times*, December 19, 1952.
2. Hall, Lawrence B. 1994. Herbert S. Gaskill, M.D., (1909-1993) [Obituary]. *International Journal of Psychoanalysis*, 75:1269-1271.

## Hanus Jiri Grosz

1. Dr. Hanus Grosz was professor of psychiatry, practicing psychiatrist. *Indianapolis Star*, September 30, 2001.

## John H. Greist

1. Dr. John Greist, 53-year psychiatrist, established lab at Methodist Hospital. *Indianapolis Star*, March 7, 1994.

## Charles Keith Hepburn

1. Dr. Charles Hepburn dies; was neurologist. *Indianapolis Star*, March 30, 1970.

## Frank Frazier Hutchins

1. Dr. F.F. Hutchins dies in hospital. *Indianapolis Star*, September 23, 1942.

## Donald H. Jolly

1. Muscatatuck State Hospital. *Muscatatuck Mirror*, February 1967.
2. Muscatatuck State Hospital. *Muscatatuck Mirror*, March 1967.

## Jefferson F. Klepfer

1. Deza, Ernest C. Forum: The reader's corner. *Indianapolis Star Magazine.* June 20, 1976, p. 23.
2. Dr. Jeffersoon Klepfer dies; Richmond State Hospital head. *Indianapolis Star*, March 1, 1976.

## Helen P. Langner

1. Curtis, John. Women in medicine: A life of engagement. *Yale Magazine*, Summer, 1998.

## John Augustus Larson

1. Belles, Dale. Longcliff triples its staff and becomes a hospital, not merely just an institution. With new superintendent it revolutionizes old procedure. *Logansport Pharos Tribune*, April 6, 1950.
2. Dr. J.A. Larson dies; developed polygraph test. *Indianapolis Times*, September 23, 1965.
3. Mikels, Donna. Uses of lie detector dismay its inventor. *Indianapolis Times*, November 27, 1949.
4. Milestones: October 1, 1965. *Time Magazine*, October 1, 1965.
5. Wilson, John V. Logansport Hospital chief fired. Dr. Morgan speedily names successor to Supt. Larson. Inefficiency, mismanagement, difficulty with staff charged; Southworth takes over. *Indianapolis Times*, September 29, 1955.

## Earl W. Mericle

1. Dr. Earl W. Mericle dies: Was in neuro-psychiatry. *Indianapolis Star*, March 8, 1979.

## Donald Floyd Moore

1. Dr. Donald F. Moore: Hoosier in profile. *Indianapolis Star Magazine*, March 2, 1975, pp. 39-45.
2. Dr. Donald Floyd Moore. [Obituary] *Indianapolis Star*, September 12, 1999.

3. Dr. Donald Moore assumes post of medical director. *The Courier.* Indianapolis, Indiana: Larue D. Carter Memorial Hospital, October 17, 1955.

4. Schmetzer, Alan, Small, Joyce and Small, Iver. 2009. Donald Floyd Moore, M.D. and other superintendents of Carter Hospital – A brief history. Spectrum [Indiana Psychiatric Society], 44(6):5,8.

## Margaret Elaine Morgan

1. Dr. Morgan tagged for health post. *Indianapolis Star*, May 13, 1953.

2. Leibowitz, Irving. Dr. Morgan, "cover girl." *Indianapolis Times*, August 5, 1955.

3. Medicine: Pride of Indiana. *Time*, October 18, 1954.

4. Zimmerman, Gereon. Psychiatrist on the spot: Indiana's governor promised the voters a cleanup of mental-health institutions. Then he handed the broom to Dr. Morgan. *Look*, March 31, 1955, pp. 43-44.

5. Dr. Margaret Morgan. *Vogue*, February 1, 1955, p. 166.

6. Dr. Margaret E. Morgan. [Obituary] *Scottsburg Giveaway*, January 14, 2004.

## William E. Murray

1. Dr. William Murray initiated mental health outreach efforts. [Obituary] *Indianapolis Star*, July 17, 1998.

## Juul C. Nielsen

1. Dr. Juul C. Nielsen to head new Carter Hospital. *Indianapolis Star*, March 25, 1951.

2. Nielsen, Juul C. 1952. Another milestone. *Monthly Bulletin of the Indiana State Board of Health*, 40(9):195-199.

## John I. Nurnberger, Sr.

1. Dr. John I. Nurnberger had been head of psychiatry at IU School of Medicine. *Indianapolis Star*, June 12, 2001.

2. I.U. Psychiatry chief selected. *Indianapolis News*, October 20, 1955.

## Philip B. Reed

1. Dr. Philip Reed III, 90, practiced neuropsychiatry. *Indianapolis Star*, March 14, 1997.
2. Reed, Philip. Curriculum vitae.

## Nancy C. A. Roeske

1. Dr. Nancy Roeske rites set; professor of psychiatry. *Indianapolis Star*, April 26, 1986.
2. Nurnberger, John I., Hendrie, Hugh C., Simmons, James E. Nancy Roeske Memorial Resolution. Indianapolis, Indiana: Indiana University School of Medicine, 1986.
3. Roeske, Nancy A. and Assue, Clare M. (Eds.) *Examination of the Personality*. Indiana University School of Medicine: Indianapolis, Indiana, 1969.

## William Leland Sharp

1. Clark, Gloria. Reflecting on the treatment of mental illness. *Anderson Sunday Herald*, November 23, 1986.
2. Dr. William L. Sharp. [Obituary] *Anderson Herald-Bulletin*, September 26, 1994.
3. William L. Sharp. Curriculum vitae.

## Patricia Haig Sharpley

1. Patricia Sharpley was chief of hospitals' adult services. *Indianapolis Star*, May 18, 1997.

## James E. Simmons

1. Blix, Suzanne. James E. Simmons Memorial Resolution. Indianapolis, Indiana: Indiana University School of Medicine, 1998.
2. Dr. James Simmons, psychiatry professor. [Obituary] *Indianapolis Star*, August 31, 1998.

3. James E. Simmons. *Psychiatric examination of children.* Philadelphia: Lea & Febiger, 1969.

## E. Rogers Smith

1. E. Rogers Smith, neurologist dies. *Indianapolis Star,* July 3, 1972.

## William C. Strang

1. Dr. William C. Strang, 89, was psychiatrist, taught at IU. *Indianapolis Star,* October 5, 2002.

## Wallace Van Den Bosch

1. Beatty can't become prison, says doctor. *Indianapolis News,* September 29, 1956.
2. Wallace Van Den Bosch. [Obituary] *Lafayette Journal and Courier,* January 1, 2006.

## Walter Crowe VanNuys

1. Dr. W. C. VanNuys, native of Waveland, dies at Dayton, Ohio. *Crawfordsville Journal Review,* December 12, 1955.
2. Kellum, Robert W. State Village for Epileptics monument to humane spirit. *Indianapolis Star,* June 12, 1948.

## George C. Weinland

1. Dr. George Weinland. [Obituary] *Columbus Republic,* September 10, 2004.

## Clifford L. Williams

1. Dr. C.L. Williams named chief of central hospital. *Indianapolis Star,* February 22, 1952.
2. Dr. Williams dies; Former hospital head. *Indianapolis Star,* October 2, 1967.
3. Dr. Williams heads mental health council. *Indianapolis Star,* December 28, 1945.

4. Power, Fremont. A big man copes with mental ills. *Indianapolis News*, January 26, 1966.

## James J. Wright

1. Dr. James J. Wright was psychiatrist, past director of mental health center. *Indianapolis Star*, April 22, 2001.
2. Schmetzer, Alan D., Butler, Nancy E., McDougle, Christopher and Rau, N. Lela. Memorial resolution on behalf of James J. Wright, Assistant Professor Emeritus of psychiatry at Indiana University School of Medicine. Indianapolis, Indiana: Indiana University School of Medicine, September 6, 2001.

## Chapter 14 Notable Non Psychiatrists from Indiana

### Morris Herman Aprison

1. Dr. Morris Aprison. [Obituary] *Indianapolis Star*, December 4, 2007.

### Malcolm B. Ballinger

1. Ballinger, Malcolm B. My interest in pastoral psychology. Ohio Valley Chapter of the College of Pastoral Supervision and Psychotherapy, Inc. http:/cpspovalley.org//news/articles/p counseling.pdf
2. Malcolm B. Ballinger. [Obituary] *Indianapolis Star*, February 1, 2007.

### Norman Madrid Beatty

1. Dr. Beatty, fighter for mentally ill is dead. *Indianapolis News*, December 6, 1948.
2. Inside Indianapolis, Hoosier profile, Norman Madrid Beatty. *Indianapolis Times*, May 24, 1947.
3. Norman M. Beatty, physician. Indianapolis, Indiana: Citizens Historical Association: January 7, 1939.

## Walter L. Bruetsch

1.  Holmes, Lelia. Psychiatric trailblazer recalls state's first medical research. *Indianapolis Star*, June 18, 1967.
2.  King, Lucy Jane. 2000. The best possible means of benefiting the incurable: Walter Bruetsch and the malaria treatment of paresis. *Annals of Clinical Psychiatry*, 12:197-203.
3.  Services held for research pathologist Dr. W.L. Bruetsch. *Indianapolis Star*, February 4, 1977.

## Ezra Vernon Hahn

1.  Dr. E. Vernon Hahn, neurosurgeon, dies. *Indianapolis Star*, October 17, 1959.
2.  E. Vernon Hahn, surgeon. Citizens Historical Association, December 31, 1938.

## Alfred Charles Kinsey

1.  Medicine: Dr. Kinsey of Bloomington. *Time Magazine*, January 5, 1948.
2.  Medicine: 5940 women. *Time Magazine*, August 24, 19538.
3.  Medicine: How men behave. *Time Magazine*, January 5, 1948.
4.  Kinsey, Alfred C., Pomeroy, Wardell B., Martin, Clyde E. *Sexual Behavior in the Human Male*. Philadelphia, Pennsylvania: W.B. Saunders, 1948.
5.  Kinsey, Alfred C., Pomeroy, Wardell B., Martin, Clyde E, and Gebhard, Paul. "*Sexual Behavior in the Human Female*. Philadelphia, Pennsylvania: W.B. Saunders, 1953.

## Eugene E. Levitt

1.  Bernard Lubin and William George McAdoo. 1997. Eugene E. Levitt (1921-1995). [Obituary] *American Psychologist*, 52:471.

## Carrie Lively

1.  Lively, Carrie E. 1983. Reminiscences of a state mental hospital attendant. *Indiana Medical History Quarterly*, 11(3):13-22.

## Victor Milstein

1. Dr. Victor Milstein. [Obituary] *Indianapolis Star*, April 10, 2009.

## Ruth Rogers

1. Post, Margaret Moore. She helps others. *Indianapolis News*, March 30, 1982.
2. Weinberg, Irene. Alumni profiles: Ruth Rogers. Indiana University School of Social Work Alumni Association. http://alumni.iupui.edu/associations/socialwork/profiles/rogers.html

## Norman Skole

1. Norman Skole [Obituary] *Indianapolis Star*, November 2, 2007.

## Samuel E. Smith

1. Dr. Samuel E. Smith: An appreciation. *Supplement to the thirty ninth annual report of the Richmond State Hospital*. Richmond, Indiana: Easthaven Press, 1940.
2. Dr. S.E. Smith, I.U. provost, dies: Insanity authority is heart attack victim – ill five months. *Indianapolis Star*, May 30, 1928.
3. Dr. S.E. Smith rites to be held Saturday. Expert on insanity victim of heart disease at home. Was nationally known. *Indianapolis News*, May 30, 1928.

# Chapter 15 Laws

## Selected Mental Health Laws in Indiana

1. Ewbank, Louis B. and Riker, Dorothy L. (Eds.) An act concerning insane persons. *The laws of Indiana Territory, 1809-1816*. Indianapolis, Indiana: Indiana Historical Bureau, 1934, pp. 650-652.

2.  Indiana General Assembly. *Laws of the state of Indiana passed and published by the second session of the General Assembly.* Corydon, Indiana: A & J Brandon, printer, 1818, pp. 331-332.

3.  Indiana General Assembly. *Laws of a general nature passed at the twenty-fourth session of the General Assembly of the state of Indiana commenced at Indianapolis on Monday the second day of December, 1939.* Indianapolis, Indiana: J. Livingston, printer, 1840, pp. 72.

4.  Indiana General Assembly. An act to provide for the procuring of a suitable site for the erection of a State Lunatic Asylum. *General laws of the state of Indiana passed at the twenty-ninth session of the General Assembly begun on the first Monday in December, 1844.* Indianapolis, Indiana: J.P. Chapman, state printer, 1845, pp. 58-59.

5.  Indiana General Assembly. An act authorizing the erection of suitable buildings for the use of the Indiana Hospital for the Insane. *General laws of the state of Indiana passed at the thirtieth session of the General Assembly begun on the first Monday in December, 1845.* Indianapolis, Indiana: J.P. Chapman, state printer, 1846, pp. 116-118.

6.  Indiana General Assembly. An act to provide for the confinement of persons insane and dangerous when suffered to run at large and for the compensation of him to whom the custody of such insane person is committed. *Laws of the state of Indiana passed at the thirty-eighth session of the General Assembly.* Indianapolis, Indiana: Austin H. Brown, printer, 1855, pp. 131-136.

7.  Indiana General Assembly. An act regulating sanity inquests, and the committal of insane persons to hospitals for the insane, and their discharge therefrom. *Laws of the state of Indiana passed at the fifty-second regular session of the General Assembly.* Indianapolis, Indiana: Carlon & Hollenbeck, printer, 1881, pp. 545-555.

8.  Indiana General Assembly. An act providing for the location of additional hospitals for the insane, and providing management thereof. *Laws of the state of Indiana passed at the fifty-third regular session of the General Assembly.* Indianapolis, Indiana: William B. Buford, printer 1883, pp. 164-168.

9. Indiana General Assembly. An act regulating sanity inquests, and the committal of insane persons to hospitals for the insane, and their discharge therefrom. *Laws of the state of Indiana passed at the fifty-sixth regular session of the General Assembly.* Indianapolis, Indiana: William B. Buford, printer, 1889, pp. 391-395.

10. Indiana General Assembly. An act concerning the disposition and custody of persons who become insane after conviction for crime, providing how such insanity shall be determined, and providing by whom the costs and expenses of such proceeding may be paid. *Laws of the state of Indiana passed at the sixty-fourth regular session of the General Assembly.* Indianapolis, Indiana: William B. Buford, printer, 1905, pp. 174-175.

11. Indiana General Assembly. An act authorizing and providing for the establishment of a hospital for insane criminals" as a part of the 'Indiana State Prison,' making appropriations therefore, providing for its government and maintenance, defining the manner of holding insanity inquests in cases of conviction alleged to be insane and for their transfer or discharge, repealing all laws in conflict and declaring an emergency." *Laws of the state of Indiana passed at the sixty-sixth regular session of the General Assembly.* Indianapolis, Indiana: William B. Buford, printer, 1909, pp. 202-208.

12. Indiana General Assembly. An act to rename the hospitals for the insane, prescribing the rights, powers and duties of such hospitals as a result of the change in the names and providing for the conclusion of proceedings begun under or by the name by which such hospitals were formerly known. *Laws of the state of Indiana passed at the seventy-fifth regular session of the General Assembly.* Indianapolis, Indiana: William B. Buford, printer, 1927, pp. 128-131.

13. Indiana General Assembly. *Acts of 1945 of the Indiana General Assembly.* Indianapolis, Indiana, Chapter 335, Section 8, Paragraph 5.

14. Indiana General Assembly. An act defining criminal sexual psychopathic persons, providing a lawful procedure in adjudging a person to be a criminal sexual psychopathic person, giving courts having general jurisdiction of criminal cases jurisdiction thereof, providing for their commitment and confinement to

suitable institutions for their care and treatment, their parole and discharge therefrom, the apprehension and return of escaped criminal sexual psychopathic persons, providing for tome and place of trial, providing for appeals therefrom, and declaring an emergency. *Laws of the state of Indiana passed at the eighty-sixth regular session of the Indiana General Assembly.* Indianapolis, Indiana: Bookwalter Company, 1945, pp. 1569-1570.

15. Indiana General Assembly. An act concerning the discharge of patients from the psychiatric hospitals of this state, prescribing a procedure therefore, and prescribing a procedure for the restoration of the civil rights of patients who are discharged from psychiatric hospitals. *Laws of the state of Indiana passed at the eighty-sixth regular session of the Indiana General Assembly.* Indianapolis, Indiana: Bookwalter Company, 1945, p. 1064.

16. Indiana General Assembly. An act prescribing the proceedings for the admission of mentally ill persons to psychiatric hospitals; and prescribing penalties. *Laws of the state of Indiana passed at the eighty-sixth regular session of the Indiana General Assembly.* Indianapolis, Indiana: Bookwalter Company, 1957, pp. 1046-1062.

## Eugenics

1. Lantzer, Jason S. and Stern, Alexandra Minna. 2007. Building a fit society: Indiana's eugenics crusaders. *Traces of Indiana and Midwestern History*, 19(1):4-11.

2. Osgood, Robert L. 2001. The menace of the feebleminded: George Bliss, Amos Butler, and the Indiana Committee on Mental Defectives. *Indiana Magazine of History*, 98:253-277.

3. The future care of the feeble-minded. June 1916. *Indiana Bulletin of Charities and Corrections.*

4. Indiana General Assembly. An act to provide for the sexual sterilization of inmates at state institutions in certain cases. *Laws of the state of Indiana passed at the seventy-fifth regular session of the General Assembly.* Indianapolis, Indiana: William B. Buford, 1927, pp. 713-717.

5. Kaelber, Lutz. Eugenics, Compulsory sterilization in 50 American states, Indiana. University of Vermont. http://www.uvm.edu/~lkaelber/eugenics/IN/IN.html

6. Stern, Alexandra Minna. 2007. "We cannot make a silk pure out of a sow's ear": Eugenics in the Hoosier heartland. *Indiana Magazine of History*, 103(3):3-38.

## Preliminary Mental Examination

1. Indiana General Assembly. Mental examination preliminary to sanity inquest provided for. *Laws of the state of Indiana, Regular Session 84th General Assembly*. Indianapolis, Indiana: C.E. Pauley [Printer], 1945, pp. 33-38.

## Mental Health Court:

1. Bowman, Elizabeth S. Indiana's Most Unique Court. *Indiana Psychiatric Society Newsletter*, July 1986.

## Landmark Indiana Cases

1. Jackson v Indiana, 406 U.S. 715 (1972)
2. Burns v Reed, 500 U.S. 478 (1991)
3. Indiana v Edwards, 554 USSC (2008)
4. Benitz, Christopher T. and Chamberlain, John. 2008. Competency to stand trial and to waive the sixth amendment right to self-representation. *Journal of the American Academy of Psychiatry and the Law*, 36:261-263.
5. Morris, Douglas R. and Frierson, Richard L. 2008. Pro se competence in the aftermath of Indiana v. Edwards. *Journal of the American Academy of Psychiatry and the Law*, 36:551-557.

# Chapter 16 Cases, Famous and Infamous

## Anna Keyt Agnew

1. Agnew, Anna. *From under the cloud or personal reminiscences of insanity*. Cincinnati, Ohio: Robert C. Clarke & Co., 1886.

2. Flynn, Elizabeth. 2009. Dark clouds in the mind: An overview of mental health care in Indiana's State Hospital for the Insane. *Connections: The Hoosier Genealogist,* 49:68-75.

3. King. Lucy Jane. *The sevens steeples: Anna Agnew and the Indiana Hospital for the Insane.* Zionsville, Indiana: Guild Press/Emmis Publishing, 2002.

## Anthony G. Kiritsis

1. Comiskey, Daniel S. End of the line. *Indianapolis Monthly,* February 2007, 128-135.

2. Crime: I'll have vengeance. *Time Magazine,* February 21, 1977.

3. Stanton, Niles. The insanity case of State of Indiana v. Anthony G. Kiritsis, Marion County Superior Court 5, Indianapolis Indiana (1977). University of Maryland. http://faculty.ed.umuc.edu/~nstanton/Kiritsis.html

4. Sterne, Arthur L.. Tony Kiritsis (or testing my most famous patient). In, Arthur L. Sterne, *Things I know or think I know or thought I knew or Who knows?* Bloomington, Indiana: iUniverse, 2009, pp. 154-156.

5. Tony Kiritsis, 72, found deed of natural causes. In '77 he wired a shotgun around the neck of a mortgage company official, paraded him through downtown, kept him hostage for days. *Indianapolis Star,* January 29, 2005.

6. Hill, Kristie. Associated Press, February 8, 1977.

7. Associated Press. February 10, 1977.

8. State of Indiana on the relation of Anthony G. Kiritsis v. Marion Probate Court and the Honorable Victor S. Pfau, Judge. No. 678S108 Supreme Court of Indiana 269 Ind. 550; 381N.E.2d 1245; 1978 Ind. LEXIS 811

9. Judge rejects Kiritsis' bid for freedom. Associated Press, December 28, 1984.

10. Richardson, Doug. Gunman in 1977 hostage drama rejects guardianship offer. Associated Press, December 8, 1987.

11. Huddleston, Susan. Free after nearly 11 years inside institutions for holding businessman. Associated Press, January 16, 1988.

12. Hostage-taker Kiritsis seeks billions for the 11 years he was confined. Associated Press, January 3, 1990.

## Maude Ott

1. Coons, Philip M. 2009. History of psychiatry in Indiana: Arsons at Evansville State Hospital and Logansport State Hospital: Who done it? Spectrum [Indiana Psychiatric Society], 44(6): 4,6.
2. Coons, Philip M. 2008. History of psychiatry in Indiana: Evansville State Hospital Fire. *Spectrum* [Indiana Psychiatric Society], 44(4):3.
3. Arrest couple in hospital fire: Woman attendant accused of arson, husband also held. *Logansport Pharos Tribune*, February 29, 1944.
4. Investigate fires at state hospital: Officers from state police headquarters and state fire marshal's office launch inquiry. *Logansport Pharos Tribune*, February 25, 1944.
5. Aleen Ott found unconscious in her cell at jail. *Logansport Pharos Tribune*, March 1, 1944.
6. Condition of Aleen Ott accused of hospital fires still serious. *Logansport Pharos Tribune*, March 3, 1944.
7. Probe arson mystery angles: Aleen Ott still remains in coma. *Logansport Pharos Tribune*, March 4, 1944.
8. Alleged arsonist regaining consciousness: Reiterates her threats to end life. *Logansport Pharos Tribune*, March 6, 1944.
9. Man accuses wife of 3 state hospital fires: Fatal blaze in Evansville traced to aid. *Indianapolis Star*, March 2, 1944.
10. James Ott's arson statement. *Logansport Pharos Tribune*, March 2, 1944, pp. 1,11.
11. Find Aleen Ott former mental patient: Authorities making check of past life. *Logansport Pharos Tribune*, March 9, 1944.
12. Await word on past life of Mrs. Ott. *Logansport Pharos Tribune*, March 10, 1944.
13. Mrs. Ott confesses Birdseye blaze: Set house afire to get insurance. *Logansport Pharos Tribune*, March 13, 1944.
14. Sentence Mrs. Ott for arson: Enters guilty plea in hospital blaze; meted one to ten years. *Logansport Pharos Tribune*, March 14, 1944.

15. Ott to face charge in home fire. *Logansport Pharos Tribune*, March 15, 1944.

16. Mrs. Ott kept manacled in cell: Arsonist may be taken to mental institution. *Indianapolis News*, June 6, 1944.

17. Mrs. Maude Lucas Ott, accused arsonist, is patient at hospital. *Logansport Pharos Tribune*, September 8, 1944.

18. Fraud charge filed against James Ott, 57. *Logansport Pharos Tribune*, March 18, 1944.

19. Hospital arsonist dies. *Logansport Pharos Tribune*, February 2, 1949.

### Albert Thayer

1. Albert Thayer, Civil War veteran, is dead, prominent in early life of Indianapolis, active as businessman. Indiana Commission on Public Records. http://www.in.gov/icpr/images/csh_obt.jpg

2. Thayer, Albert. Indiana crazy house. Indianapolis, Indiana: Albert Thayer.

3. Thayer, Albert. The rough diamond. Indianapolis, Indiana: Albert Thayer, January 1, 1886.

### John Zwara

1. Bonsett, Charles S. 1973. John Zwara. *Indiana Medical History Quarterly*, 1(1):3-5

2. Perry, Rachel Berenson. Summer 2005. John Zwara: The wandering artist. *Traces*, pp. 6-15.

3. John Zwara (1880-1951). Fine Arts Trader. http://fineartstrader.com/john_zwara.htm

4. Berry, S.L.. Former Central State site showcases works by Depression-era homeless painter Zwara. *Indianapolis Star*, July 19, 2005.

## Afterword

1. Lamb, H. Richard and Weinberger, Linda E. 1998. Persons with severe mental illness in jails and prisons: A review. *Psychiatric Services*, 49:483-492.

2.  Torrey, E. Fuller. 1995. Editorial: Jails and prisons – America's new mental hospitals. *American Journal of Public Health*, 85:1612-1613.

3.  Torrey, E. Fuller, Kennard, Aaron D, Eslinger, Don, et al. More mentally ill persons are in jails and prisons than hospitals: A survey of the states. Arlington, Virginia: Treatment Advocacy Center, May 2010.

4.  Parker, George F. 2009. Impact of a mental health training course for correctional officers on a special housing unit. *Psychiatric Services*, 60:640-645.

5.  Indiana Division of Mental Health and Addictions. State operated facilities transition plan. Indiana Division of Mental Health and Addictions. http://www.in.gov/fssa/dmha/files/ State_Operated_Facilities_Transition_Plan_-_7-2010.pdf

# About the Authors

**Philip M. Coons, M.D.:**

Dr. Coons is Professor Emeritus of Psychiatry at Indiana University School of Medicine in Indianapolis, Indiana. He is boarded in General Psychiatry (1976) with added qualifications in Forensic Psychiatry (1999) by the American Board of Psychiatry and Neurology.

A past president and fellow of the International Society for the Study of Trauma and Dissociation, Dr. Coons has received both of their prestigious Morton Prince and Cornelia Wilbur awards. Dr. Coons is past president of the Indiana Psychiatric Society and distinguished life fellow in the American Psychiatric Association. He is a member of the Indiana Psychiatric Society, American Psychiatric Association, International Society for the Study of Trauma and Dissociation, and the American Academy of Psychiatry and the Law. He is associate editor emeritus of the *Journal of Trauma and Dissociation*.

Dr. Coons' research interests include dissociative disorders and dissociative identity disorder. He has published numerous scientific articles and book chapters on dissociation. He is internationally recognized for his expertise on dissociation and has contributed to the development of the dissociative disorders sections of both the *International Classification of Diseases* and the *Diagnostic and Statistical Manual of Mental Disorders*.

Currently Dr. Coons' main clinical activity is the practice of forensic psychiatry.

## Elizabeth S. Bowman, M.D.:

Psychiatrist Elizabeth Bowman is currently Adjunct Professor of Neurology, the consulting psychiatrist for the Adult Epilepsy Program at Indiana University School of Medicine, and maintains a part-time private practice in Indianapolis, Indiana. She formerly was Professor of Psychiatry at Indiana University School of Medicine. Her academic interests include psychological conversion seizures, the dissociative disorders, and the religious and spiritual aspects of mental health.

Dr. Bowman is past president and fellow of the International Society for the Study of Trauma and Dissociation, from whom she received the Lifetime Achievement Award and two Distinguished Achievements Awards. She is also past president of the Indiana Psychiatric Society and a distinguished fellow in the American Psychiatric Association from whom she received the prestigious Oskar Pfister Award for work integrating religion and psychiatry. She is founding Editor Emerita of the *Journal of Trauma and Dissociation*. She is author of numerous scientific articles and book chapters on dissociative disorders, conversion seizures, and religious/spiritual aspects of psychiatry. She holds a Master of Sacred Theology degree from Christian Theological Seminary in Indianapolis.

# Appendix A

# Interview with John Greist, M.D.

Dr. Griest was interviewed at home at 4343 N. Washington Boulevard, Indianapolis, Indiana by Elizabeth Bowman, M.D., on August 21, 1986.

Indiana University School of Medicine was formed by the merger of several medical schools in Indiana. Dr. C.P. Emerson was brought from Johns Hopkins, where he had studied under Sir William Osler, to form the school. Dr. Willis Gatch was brought from St. Louis to head the Department of Surgery. Dr. Gatch was made Professor of Surgical Pathology and Dr. John Oliver took over surgery.

In the early years, the school had few full-time paid professors and most of the faculty was volunteer or part-time. Dr. Emerson brought Osler's emphasis on bedside teaching and clinical excellence to Indiana University, along with Osler's grasp of emotional factors in physical illness. The pattern of Johns Hopkins medicine was that of the internist being the leading figure, doing his or her own neurology and psychiatry. Neither specialty was particularly developed at that point. Neurology developed more rapidly here that did psychiatry. Dr. Emerson could see the on-coming need for neurologists and brought in some neurologists to teach. Among those people was Dr. Albert Stern who trained in neurology in Europe. The neurologists were involved in psychiatry through the treatment of neurosyphilis, a very common illness in those days. At that time, tertiary paresis patients filled about a third of all the state hospital beds. Thus, the neurologists carried the load of psychiatry almost as an adjunct to their neurological work.

Dr. Larue Carter came in the World War I era. He was a neurologist from Westfield. After serving in WWI as a division surgeon for the 38th Division of the Indiana National Guard, he returned to Indianapolis and was associated with Dr. Stern who had founded the Norways Sanitarium in Indianapolis. Another early neuropsychiatrist who served in both World Wars was Dr. Frank Hutchins who taught in the 1920s. Dr. Irving Page, a brilliant researcher in chemistry and medicine, served on the Indiana University faculty. Dr. E. Rogers Smith, primarily a neurologist, trained at Michigan and taught at Indiana University. Dr Max Bahr was the Superintendent of Central State Hospital. At that time nearly all psychiatry was done in state hospitals. In the early 1920s there were probably not more than twenty neuropsychiatrists in private practice in Indiana. At Indiana University School of Medicine in the 1920s, the lectures in psychiatry consisted of two hours on Saturday afternoon in the senior year. Dr. Bahr's lectures consisted of classical descriptions of paresis, schizophrenia and senility.

In those days they were just beginning to get the edge on syphilis with Salversan. When Salversan was ineffective, Dr. Greist saw many Charcot joints and patients with paresis. In those days, Central State played an important role in the development of the malarial treatment for syphilis. Dr. Breutch, a fine German pathologist at Central State Hospital, worked out the mechanism by which malaria improved paretics by studying specimens from Central State patients. The 1920s were very interesting years with syphilis being attacked and fading out

It was not until the early 1930s that the Department of Psychiatry was formed from the Department of Neurology at Indiana University. Dr. Dave Boyd, a full-time faculty member in neurology and psychiatry, had built a strong course in neurology with the full support of Dr. Gatch (who replaced Emerson as I.U. Dean around 1932) who supported the teaching of neurology but was unsupportive, if not openly discouraging, of the teaching of psychiatry. The American Association of Medical Schools was surveying the functions of various schools. Dr. Frank Ebaugh, Professor of Psychiatry at Colorado and a former student of Dr. Adolph Meyer, was responsible for the survey of psychiatry teaching. His rating of Indiana University was very low and he made it clear to Dr. Gatch that if adequate courses were not organized, the university would lose some of its standing in the Association of Medical Colleges. Thus, some of the advances in neurology and psychiatry came without the blessings of Dean Gatch.

The Ebaugh review had a great influence on the teaching of psychiatry. Dr. Boyd, along with Dr. Alexander Ross, taught neurology and psychiatry. The eventual division of the two departments was an outgrowth of the growing number of doctors treating primarily psychiatric problems. Some of the neurologists were not at all happy about the division. Around 1929 or 1930 Dr. Emerson had set up a child guidance clinic in the basement of what is now Emerson Hall and brought a psychologist and social workers in to assist.

Dr. E. Vernon Hahn, a very fine neurosurgeon, was also interested in neuropsychiatry and went to the Chicago Psychoanalytic Institute for a personal analysis. He did not teach but did treat a number of psychiatric patients, especially during World War II. Dr. Philip Reed graduated from Indiana University, interned at Indianapolis City Hospital and was Assistant Superintendent of the hospital for a while. He then joined Drs. Stern and Carter at Norways until going to Philadelphia for psychiatric training. A year or two later, he was followed by Dr. Earl Mericle who became interested in psychiatry after doing a residency in surgery and becoming interested in neurosurgery. The bulk of Dr. Mericle's work was in neuropsychiatry. During WW II he was a division psychiatrist working in combat zones and earned the respect of William Menninger who headed army psychiatry.

Dr. L.H. Gilman, INPA President in 1941, was a neuropsychiatrist who did a good bit of supervising on the wards, including teaching Dr. Greist how to do his first cisternal puncture. Dr. Clifford Williams, INPA President in 1958, followed Dr. Bahr as Superintendent of Central State Hospital. He also taught psychiatry at Indiana University. Dr. Paul Williams, who was Assistant Superintendent with Dr. Williams was a very able teacher of psychiatry. Many medical students worked on the wards of Central State Hospital in those days and benefited from Dr. Williams' teaching.

Dr. Walter Breutch became INPA President in 1941 to complete the term of Dr. Gilman who died while serving as President. So during WW II, one of INPA's presidents was a German who had served on a German sub in WW I. Eventually he retired and returned to Germany.

Dr. Larue Carter and Dr. Sterne lectured to medical students. In addition to Norways Sanitarium on East 10th Street, there was the Fletcher Sanitarium on East Market Street, founded by Dr. Fletcher. It had little or no connection with the medical school and was a private sanitarium. It had three wards for mild moderate and severely ill patients, and a good hydrotherapy set-up. Both Norways and Fletcher were functioning when Dr. Greist returned to Indianapolis in 1935.

After Dr. Stern died, Dr. Carter took over Norways and was assisted by Dr. Reed who married Dr. Stern's foster daughter. Dr. Carter had hoped to make Norways function much as Menninger's did in Topeka. They were very generous and invited all the psychiatrists in town to be on their staff. A good deal of teaching took place at Norways.

Dr. Larue Carter was a natural for the position of first president of INPA. "He just stood out like Mount Olympus." Dr. E. Vernon Hahn, INPA's second president, was an exceedingly brilliant man and a good speaker. During WW II interest in psychiatry grew by leaps and bounds because of the public's exposure to war neurosis. The early INPA set up a group of public seminars in which a number of us, along with members of the clergy and some psychologists participated. Panel discussions on mental health were held and Dr. Hahn was very active in that, even though his major practice was still surgery. Those public meetings went on for at least two years and were held in the Shortridge High School auditorium.

# Appendix B

# Interview with Philip Reed, M.D.

Philip B. Reed, M.D., was interviewed at home in Cicero, Indiana by Elizabeth S. Bowman, M.D. on August 27, 1986.

The small gathering of men at French Lick in October 1937 led to the organization meeting of the Indiana Neuropsychiatric Association. The organizational meeting was in late 1938 or the spring of 1939.

Larue Carter was a father figure to most of the psychiatrists in the state in 1937. E. Rogers Smith [Rog] had much fun testifying as an expert witness and loved to mention that he was born in an insane asylum, while his father Samuel E. Smith was superintendent of Richmond State Hospital. When Rog was attending Indiana University and then the University of Michigan Medical School, Larue Carter was a house officer at Richmond State Hospital. Roger's father took a dim view of his boy drinking any alcohol so any time Rog had a bottle to bring home from school, he stashed it in Larue Carter's closet. Dr. Carter's relationship to a number of the younger psychiatrists may not have been based on such warm ties, but nonetheless, existed.

Dr. Carter was always much in favor of getting doctors together for discussions, be they social, semi-scientific, or scientific. With the growing number of doctors in the state who were inclined to place P, N, or NP after their names in the directory of the AMA, Larue Carter felt the time had come to get these people together and possibly form a state organization. That was done with that little group gathered in October 1937.

Those who attended that meeting on the wide porch with its tall cane chairs were John Hare (Superintendent of Evansville State Hospital), Murray DeArmond, Louis Potter Harshman of Fort Wayne, Keith Hepburn of Indianapolis, Rog Smith of Indianapolis, Clifford Williams of Indianapolis, and Phil Reed and possibly one or two others. We all agreed it was time for a state org to be formed.

The organizational meeting took place at Norways Sanitarium in Indianapolis the next spring or fall. Dr. Reed was at this meeting. Larue Carter was elected president and Phil Reed was elected secretary-treasurer. Larue Carter was asked to choose a committee and designate the functions of that committee as to drafting a constitution and bylaws for INPA. Reed had to resign his post before the second meeting because he entered the Graduate School of Medicine at the University of Pennsylvania in the fall of 1939 for a graduate course in neurology and psychiatry. The substance of the organizational meeting at Norways dealt largely with sharing opinions as to just what a neuropsychiatric association in Indiana might possibly do, where meetings might be held since the state is a fairly long one. Dr. Harshman was from northern Indiana and Dr. John Hare from Evansville and they needed to be accommodated. This need led years later to the break in the INPA with a separate organization being broken off to operate north of the Indiana Tollroad (The Northern Indiana Psychiatric Society).

The organizational meeting was held on the sun porch of Norways, furnished with white painted rattan furniture. It was a room that would easily accommodate thirty to thirty-five people. As it turned out, there were about fifteen people in attendance at that organizational meeting.

At the time of the organizational meeting, Irving Page was the physician in charge of the Lilly Research Ward at Indianapolis City Hospital. Dr. Page left Lilly's later and went on the Cleveland Clinic where he conducted research in the field of hypertension. On the occasion of the organizational meeting, Frank Hutchins, who was by then approaching retirement and the status of elder-statesman in the group, was a great conversationalist and not one to let the conversation pause. At the meeting, prior to it being called to order, Frank commented that he had read a most fascinating book, setting forth many new theories about the nervous system. The book was titled *The Chemistry of the Brain*. He turned to the man on his left and asked, do you know anything about it? The man on his left (Irving Page) said "Yes, I wrote it."

Irving Page may have trained at Cornell. He had a Rockefeller Fellowship in New York and came to be recognized for his work which concentrated more and more on hypertension. Since Eli Lilly was interested in developing medications for the treatment of hypertension (there was little available then), Dr. Page came to Indianapolis directly from his work as director of the Kaiser Wilhelm Institute in Berlin to develop the basic research on angiotensin.

Larue Carter was a birthright Quaker born in Westfield, Indiana, who graduated from the Westfield Friends Academy. He graduated from the Medical College of Indianapolis. He interned at Indianapolis City Hospital and went on to take a two-year internship at Philadelphia General where he became quite interested in psychiatry and neurology. He then went to Richmond State Hospital where he worked under Samuel E. Smith who was evidently the first provost of Indiana University Medical Center following his retirement from Richmond State Hospital. Larue Carter also spent a few years as a physician for a mining company in Colorado because times were hard and salaried positions paid little except for odd and unique openings such as at a mining company. Dr. Reed was not sure if this stint at the mining company was before or after Richmond State Hospital.

Larue Carter came to Indiana and opened a private practice, hoping eventually to specialize in psychiatry. He was in the Indiana National Guard and served on the Mexican border for about a year during the action directed at catching Francisco Villa in 1916. During his City Hospital training days, Larue Carter had met a nurse, Ann Gant, and saw her from time to time when he was in Indianapolis. They were married in 1916 while he was on leave from his Mexican border service. After WWI came along Larue Carter went immediately to training at Camp Shelby in Hattiesburg, Mississippi. He rose to the command of a base hospital with the rank of full colonel by the end of WWI. He returned to Indianapolis and at that time joined Dr. Albert Sterne at Norways Sanitarium in about 1919.

Norways was founded by Albert E. Stern. After Dr. Sterne died in 1932 Dr. Carter became the medical director of Norways. He remained in that position until his death in 1946 when Dr. Reed succeeded him. Norways was open sixty years and closed in 1957. Dr. Reed can only recall 2 early INPA meetings that were held at Norways. Most of the early meetings were held at the Athenaeum in Indianapolis. Dr. Reed could not recall the constitution committee for INPA since he was in Philadelphia when it was formed. By the time he returned eight months later, Dr. Earl Mericle had joined Larue Carter at Norways. He was to go for specialized training but WWII interrupted his plans and he joined the military.

Those physicians who were not serving in the military were spread pretty thin attempting to teach at the medical school, cover the City Hospital psychiatric service, take care of any of the usual charity cases elsewhere and such private practices as they had. Dave Boyd came as the first full time chairperson of psychiatry at Indiana University School of Medicine a year or two before WW II. He had a psychiatric faculty of about six or seven people when WWII began. Since Dr. Carter was severely hypertensive and was quite busy with his chief of psychiatry job at City Hospital and as Director of Norways, the faculty at the medical center was reduced during the war to two people: David Boyd and Philip Reed.

Dr. Reed:      "We were pretty busy and I was attempting to carry on at Norways and had a private practice, so I was only able to handle about a third of the work and Dave Boyd handled about two-thirds of it. There were no residents in psychiatry at that time and we worked with medical students and interns at City Hospital. The interest in psychiatry demonstrated in the military in WW II greatly aroused civilian interest and demand on the part of physicians for formal training, seminars, discussions, orientations and information. Thus, residencies were being created rather rapidly. Dave Boyd set up a residency training program at City Hospital and two of the early products of this program were Dr. Louie Nie, and Dr. DeWitt Brown. A residency program was approved by the AMA and ABPN for Norways. It trained twenty-nine residents before Norways closed in 1957. The residency was three years then. Any individual could take 1, 2, or 3 years in any one locale, but had to complete three years of residency plus two years of experience in an approved setting to be eligible for boards. Boards were entirely oral then. The ABPN was founded in 1934 and grandfathered in a number of people."

Dr. Bowman:   "What was the orientation to psychiatry in this early group that formed the INPA?"

Dr. Reed:      "It varied with the age of the men and women that characterized the earliest membership roster. The mean age was around forty-five or fifty. This pretty well threw the medical and any psychiatric training they may have had back to the pre-WWI era. The process of becoming a psychiatrist, as far as the AMA was concerned, consisted of indicating your field of interest and how you wished to be designated in the directory. (This was prior to the ABPN). At the time of the founding of INPA, the majority of the founding members were practicing both neurology and psychiatry. Only one person in Indianapolis, Dr. Alex Ross, was attempting to practice pure neurology even in the few years after WWII. But since he was associated for a few years with Dr. Roger Smith and since Dr. Smith's practice was essentially psychiatric, Dr. Ross necessarily had to see a number of psychiatric patients. As for dynamic psychiatry and its influence, Dr. Vernon Hahn, who had a surgical residency at Indiana University around the time that WWII was fomenting, took an analysis in Chicago and commuted for it. In his odd hours he assisted in neurosurgical procedures in Chicago and on this basis came back to Indianapolis not as a psychoanalyst, but as a neurosurgeon. But he had a keen interest in dynamic psychiatry. Because of our keen interest in dynamic psychiatry, we made number of trips to Topeka, Kansas and received help directly from Drs. Carl and Bill Menninger. We modeled the residency at Norways quite openly and directly after the program at Menninger's. We directed a number of psychiatrists who wished formal analytic training to Topeka or elsewhere. Dr. Vince Alig, Dr. McNamara (in Minnesota) were two of these people. There was quite a mixture of orientations in the INPA.

The first scientific sessions included Dr. Breutch's ongoing work at Central State Hospital on the malarial treatment of paresis, Norway's staff reports on what was then the only insulin coma treatment in the state for treating schizophrenia and a little later the first ECT treatment in the state which was at Norways. We also discussed what might be effective sedation for manic patients (we had no psychotropic drugs). The prolonged sleep program that was used at Presbyterian Hospital in New York and at the University of Wisconsin, we used it at Norways for manics. [We] used sodium amytal."

Dr. Bowman:    "E. Vernon Hahn was the President of INPA in 1939. Do you remember that?"

| | |
|---|---|
| Dr. Reed: | "I was gone then but was aware of his presidency. He saw a limited numbers of patients for analytic treatment even though he was primarily a neurosurgeon. |
| Dr. Bowman: | "E. Rogers Smith was president in 1940?" |
| Dr. Reed: | "He was in private practice then." |
| Dr. Bowman: | "Do you remember any other officers before WWII?" |
| Dr. Reed: | "No, I do not." |
| Dr. Bowman: | "Dr. Gilman was President in 1941. What was his first name?" |
| Dr. Reed: | "L.H. were his initials. He preferred not to reveal what they stood for and he preferred to called Toby by his friends. Otherwise, he was known as L.H. He had been an extern at Norways immediately after WWI and decided to go into psychiatry. I am not absolutely clear as to whether he had a year or more of training at Central State Hospital." |
| Dr. Bowman: | "Do you know if INPA was incorporated?" |
| Dr. Reed: | "No, I don't know." |
| Dr. Bowman: | "Was it a branch of the APA?" |
| Dr. Reed: | "It could not be at the outset because the district branches were not organized yet. INPA sent its first delegate to the APA around 1968. I was that delegate and continued to serve as the delegate from this district branch for some eight or nine years, then moved up to the regional committee, then became Vice President of the APA in 1969-70. The other Indiana people who had served as officers of the APA were: Dr. Rogers who had been the superintendent at Logansport was President of the APA possibly before it was known as the APA. Dr. Rogers was responsible for the training of E. Rogers Smith's father and E. Rogers Smith was named after Dr. Rogers. Roger's father, Dr. S.E. Smith later became Superintendent of Richmond State Hospital. S.E. Smith was a President of the APA. They called him Psycho Sam. |
| Dr. Bowman: | "Dr. Gilman's term was completed by Dr. Breutch. Dr. Gilman died while INPA President in 1941. Dr. Boyd became President in 1942. Then there are no presidents |

listed until 1947? Was this because things were so interrupted by the War?"

Dr. Reed:     I think that is correct. We had occasional informal meetings in the homes of various psychiatrists in the Indianapolis area, but there were no scientific papers, just social gatherings to keep the spirit of the psychiatric group alive.

Dr. Bowman:   "Were there notes or minutes?"

Dr. Reed:     "I cannot certify as to 1944, 1945, or 1946. I think there were formal meetings and it is even possible that officers were elected. Dr. Kissel's notes don't show anything for those years but that does not coincide with my memory. WWII was definitely long over before his notes resume. [This refers to a letter from Dr. Wesley Kissell to Dr. Nancy Roeske, dated September 11, 1981, listing what he could find of the early presidents of the INPA.] Physicians did have an allotment of gasoline and were able to get tires during the war, so that was not the problem with meeting. The problem was trying to cover all of the psychiatric business of Marion County, which the City Hospital was distinctly responsible for in those early days since there were no psychiatric beds at the University and Methodist had only a few psych beds in the basement. Norways and Fletcher's Sanitarium were both private.

Fletcher's Sanitarium was founded by Dr. William Fletcher, one of the early Superintendents of Central State Hospital. He served during the Civil War. He was a prisoner of the Confederates during part of the Civil War and shortly after his return he founded the Fletcher Sanitarium. It was still functioning when I was at my early years at Norways. Dr. Carter was acquainted with Drs. Mary and Urbanna Spink who took over after Dr. Fletcher's death. They ran the Sanitarium but were desirous of retiring and wanted someone to take over the Fletcher Sanitarium. They talked to me about it but I was too busy at Norways and ultimately the Fletchers Sanitarium became a center for the treatment of VD during WW II. After this it was razed. It was on East Market Street.

Norways was at 1820 E. 10th Street. It had the whole block. It was razed in 1957 shortly after we closed. There's a supermarket there now. We did use about a half acre of ground out there for use by the Marion County Child Guidance Clinic which operated out there until a few years ago."

Dr. Bowman:     "After the war, E. Vernon Hahn took over presidency from 1947-49. What do you recall about the meetings then?"

Dr. Reed:     "Vernon was a very well-organized person and readily accepted the scientific discipline from his earliest years. He set the post-war II example for many of the officers that followed in arranging for papers well in advance and having as many speakers as possible from out of state and elevating the tone of the psychiatric association to a fairly high scientific level. We met seven times a year, not meeting through the summer and not meeting in December. The attendance in the immediate post-World War II years was fifteen to forty, forty being the swollen number that resulted when Larue Carter Hospital came into being and at a time when Norways had seven residents. We saw to it that they attended en mass. That was the late 1940s. Of course, Larue Carter Hospital did not actually function as far as residency training was concerned until about 1950.

Larue Carter Hospital's cornerstone was laid in 1949. Dr. Carter's widow was there and Governor [Henry] Schricker. I well remember the occasion. The first Superintendent of Logansport State Hospital came from Minnesota. It was wisely decided that Larue Carter Hospital, with its over two hundred beds could only open a section at a time. It was decided that if it got up above one hundred patients in its first six months of operation, that would allow for getting the bugs out in terms of staff training. Nonetheless, by the time (two or three months later) when Larue Carter Hospital had gotten up to fifteen patients, there was one resident for each patient. The Superintendent had decided to really put an emphasis on residency training. During the first two or three months they opened only one corridor and attempted to train staff. They did not feel that staff recruited from Central State would be suitable for the kind of treatment they wanted to give at Larue Carter Hospital."

Dr. Bowman:    "Who was behind Larue Carter Hospital being built?"

Dr. Reed:    "Larue Carter was probably the driving force, but he had no idea the hospital would be named after him. He had been dead about three years when it was built. I recall the occasion of learning what name would be given the hospital. The real mover for improvement of the state mental health picture was not a psychiatrist at all, but a good friend and fellow physician of Larue Carter, Dr. Norman Beatty, who was a dermatologist. Dr. Beatty was a son-in-law of the former governor, Mr. Jackson who served back in the 1940s. Norm served on the Indiana Mental Health Council which was charged with upgrading the state mental health facilities and care generally. It was decided by that group, beginning immediately after WWII, that with the backwardness of Indiana's state psychiatric program, some catalyst was necessary and that catalyst might better serve a relatively large number of trainees who would hopefully filter out in the state system in great enough numbers to upgrade care. Meanwhile, in this model hospital [Larue Carter Hospital], a certain number of patients who would be screened for admission that they might better serve as teaching cases, would be admitted. With a view to consolidating the training, it was decided the hospital would be built as close as possible to Indiana University Medical Center.

Back to the breaking of the news about the naming of Larue Carter Hospital, Norm Beatty had a myocardial infarction and Reed went out to Robert Long Hospital to call on him. He seemed to be responding to the then relatively simple treatment of giving oxygen to coronary patients. He looked good but his EKG didn't look good. He indicated to me in a phone conference which was held with him as the Indiana Mental Health Conference proceeded that the hospital would be named Larue Carter Hospital. The next day as I visited him he indicated in a rather matter of fact tone that he was not going to get well. I differed mildly with him and told him all the signs were good but he seemed to know better than I did because he died within seventy-two hours. The second hospital built was then named the Norman Beatty Hospital.

Dr. Juul Nielsen was the first superintendent of Larue Carter Hospital. Dr. Nielsen attempted to tie Larue Carter Hospital intimately with the psychiatric community. Those of us who had lived through the years of planning Larue Carter Hospital saw it as serving as a prototype for teaching and ultimately for service in all the state hospitals. We did not feel its activities and interests should be co-mingled with private psychiatry. Dr. Nielsen saw it somewhat differently and asked all the members of the Neuropsychiatric Society, at least those in the central portion of the state, attend a meeting in his apartment at Larue Carter Hospital, which we did. At that time he proposed that since Larue Carter Hospital had a number of empty beds, it would serve the training purposes of his rather large residency staff if those of us in private psychiatry would consider housing some of our private patients at Larue Carter Hospital, using them as teaching patients. The consensus, which was rather overwhelming, ran contrary to Dr. Nielsen's ideas. So his suggestion was never put into effect.

Dr. Bowman:    "You were president of INPA from 1950-51. Murray DeArmond preceded you and John Greist followed you. What was happening in INPA during the time you were president?"

Dr. Reed:    "By 1950 most of the membership had pretty well catalogued what could or could not be done with insulin coma, electroconvulsive therapy for schizophrenics. Insulin coma was gradually being phased out. Psychotropic medication had not yet come along and we had distinct limitations in the treatment of depression, manics and hypomanics. Fortunately, true mania, for reasons of which I am not aware, has statistically tended to go out of style in the last hundred years. We did not see the number of acute severe manias that Larue Carter saw in his early psychiatric days and he recalled the reminiscences of Sam Smith which indicated that there had been a diminution in the incidence of acute mania. We were fortunate in that regard."

Dr. Bowman: "The 1950-51 period was a rather solid time for the members working together on the rather single purpose of upgrading psychiatric care in the state in both public and private facilities. Was INPA politically active?"

Dr. Reed: "I would prefer to think that I was never particularly politically active but happened to come along at the right place, the right time and having the right experience and got a certain job. I am thinking of the State Medical Association Grievance Committee. My good friend and colleague, Earl Mericle had become President of the State Medical Association and he felt strongly that a psychiatrist should be on the grievance committee. He was aware that the majority of problem doctors had emotional problems, to put it mildly. So I started serving and I was elected chairman the third year I was on in, and I was chairman for nine terms. I prefer to think of it as coincidence rather than political activity. This committee split the impaired physicians committee off of it and it was free to deal with complaints on the more technical aspects of medicine.

INPA was sporadically active politically. When it was felt that we badly needed added beds in the state mental hospital system, we became active. As usual, organizations do not act as monoliths, but you have four or five people who are movers and six or eight people who will help them move. This is the way pressure was put on the state legislators and others that resulted in the plans led chiefly through Norman Beatty to get two new state hospitals. Norman Beatty regularly attended INPA meetings to get a feeling what the psychiatrists in the state wanted and needed to get done. It was left up to him to do the lobbying and he was a very powerful one-man lobbying committee. So getting two new state hospitals was a big accomplishment of those years.

Dr. Bowman: "I can't help but think that some of the planning must have gone on during those years for which we have no list of officers."

Dr. Reed: "Yes. We had many meetings at Larue Carter's home with Norm Beatty and four or five others. They were simply strategy meetings in terms of who was to see who and what was our goal and how were we going to present it to get these hospitals built. Larue Carter lived at 4280 N. Meridian. It's a small gray cottage. He lived next door to his old schoolmate and lifetime friend, John Cunningham, who lived on the corner. He was at that time regarded by many as the dean of Indiana medicine doctors. Right next door to John Cunningham on 43rd Street was Oscar Ritchey. Immediately south of Dr. Carter was the residence of Booth Tarkington who is said to have written in a letter to a friend, "I sleep peacefully at night because three of Indiana's better physicians' homes can be seen from my bedroom window. I hope at least one of them still makes house calls!""

Dr. Bowman: "Who else came to the meetings at Larue Carter's house?"

Dr. Reed: "Myself, Norm Beatty, Earl Mericle, Larue Carter. Norm convinced the legislature through non-physicians. He had apparently picked up enough politics from his father-in-law so that he could button-hole legislators out in the corridor so that they would pledge that they were going to go out on that floor and present something. He was very persuasive. He didn't twist wrists but he certainly tweaked their cortices."

Dr. Bowman: "You are the adopted son of Larue Carter?"

Dr. Reed: "I wasn't raised by him. My father died just before I graduated from high school. My mother died when I was a resident in medicine at City Hospital in 1932. I was not at Norways until 1934. I had married Genevieve

Pickrell who was the foster daughter of Albert Stern. Her father had died in 1932. Dr. Carter was very fond of Genevieve and over time we developed a very fond relationship. We worked together for over twelve years before his death. He had discussed with Ann Carter the fact that they were childless, that Genevieve's mother wouldn't live forever, and she might die leaving both of us without parents, so what did Ann think about adopting both of us? Sadly Dr. Carter died in January of 1946. He had seen most of "his boys" come home from service and he was very proud of them. They had gone to an attorney and had all of this drawn up during Larue Carter's lifetime. Posthumously Ann Carter adopted both of us."

Dr. Reed's vital statistics:

I went to Indiana University for college and worked my way for the most part and graduated in 1928 with a B.S. in anatomy. I got my M.D. in 1930 from Indiana University. I was the dog surgery assistant while I was in school and got interested in some research in dog surgery that was going on then. I was an intern and resident in medicine at City Hospital and worked on weekends over at the dog surgery department at Indiana University doing research. With two years of that I picked up my cum laude for research on those topics. I was at City Hospital in 1932. From mid-1932 to 1933 I was Assistant Superintendent at City Hospital. I had a fellowship lined up at Mayo Clinic in internal medicine and I was planning to leave in July 1932 to begin that three-year fellowship when Jess Martin, the Assistant Superintendent died. Charlie Meyers, who had just become the Superintendent of City Hospital four months before, asked me to stay on as Assistant Superintendent. At that time the Assistant Superintendent was in charge of the psychiatric service. So I combined that and made it a psychiatric residency with his approval and was Assistant Superintendent for a year and a half. Then I started for the Mayo Clinic. I had been working about sixteen hours a day. At Mayo they found an apical scar and I took a three month leave of absence in Florida and gained some weight but then I went fishing and got sunburned and the TB flared again and I was on a rest program for about six months. I decided I didn't want to go into internal medicine and take coronary calls in the middle of the night, so I decided to go into psychiatry. I went back to Indiana, joined Norways and then went in 1938 for nine months training at the University of Pennsylvania and got board certified [both neurology and psychiatry] while I was still there."

# Appendix C

## Presidents of the Indiana Neuropsychiatric Association & Indiana Psychiatric Society

The following represents an almost complete listing of the presidents of the Indiana Neuropsychiatric Association & Indiana Psychiatric Society.

Indiana Neuropsychiatric Association

| | |
|---|---|
| Larue D. Carter | 1938 |
| E. Vernon Hahn | 1939 |
| E. Rogers Smith | 1940 |
| L. H. Gilman | 1941 |
| Walter Breutsch | 1941 |
| David Boyd | 1942 |
| INPA Inactive | 1943-1946 |
| E. Vernon Hahn | 1947-1949 |
| A. Murray DeArmond | 1949-1950 |
| Philip B. Reed | 1950-1951 |
| John H. Greist | 1951-1953 |
| E. Rogers Smith | 1953-1955 |
| H. Carter Dunstone | 1955-1956 |
| Charles K. Hepburn | 1956-1957 |
| Louis W. Nie | 1957-1958 |
| Clifford L. Williams | 1958-1959 |
| Alexander Ross | 1959-1960 |
| Eldred Hardtke | 1960-1961 |
| George Rader | 1961-1962 |
| Paul Merrell | 1962-1963 |

| | |
|---|---|
| Dwight W. Schuster | 1963-1964 |
| Ronald D. Hull | 1964-1965 |

Indiana Psychiatric Association Presidents

| | |
|---|---|
| DeWitt Brown | 1965-1966 |
| Donald F. Moore | 1966-1967 |
| Gordon T. Brown | 1967-1968 |
| Robert O. Bill | 1968-1969 |
| John I. Nurnberger, Sr. | 1969-1970 |
| Ivan F. Bennett | 1970-1971 |
| John E. Kooiker | 1971-1972 |
| Wesley A. Kissell | 1972-1973 |
| Wallace R. Van Den Bosch | 1973-1974 |
| Gene E. Lynn | 1974-1975 |
| Iver F. Small | 1975-1976 |
| Robert E. Snodgrass | 1976-1977 |
| Richard N. French, Jr. | 1977-1978 |
| Philip P. Morton | 1978-1979 |
| Richard F. Rahdert | 1979-1980 |
| Sherman G. Franz | 1980-1981 |
| Nancy C. A. Roeske | 1981-1982 |
| | 1982-1983 |
| Dwight W. Schuster | 1983-1984 |
| Philip M. Coons | 1984-1985 |
| William Shriner | 1985-1986 |
| Andrew L. Morrison | 1986-1987 |
| Patricia H. Sharpley | 1987-1988 |
| Joel H. Griffith | 1988-1989 |
| Alan D. Schmetzer | 1989-1990 |
| John Yarling | 1990-1991 |
| Marvin J. Miller | 1991-1992 |
| Jon W. Holdred | 1992-1993 |
| Elizabeth S. Bowman | 1993-1994 |
| John J. Wernert | 1994-1995 |
| Steve R. Dunlap | 1995-1996 |
| David R. Diaz | 1996-1997 |
| Alan D. Schmetzer | 1997-1998 |
| John L. Yarling | 1998-1999 |

| | |
|---|---|
| Kenneth N. Weisert | 1999-2000 |
| Jeffrey J. Kellams | 2000-2001 |
| Jeffrey J. Kellams | 2001-2002 |
| Steve Nelson, Steve Fekete | 2002-2003 |
| Steve A. Fekete | 2003-2004 |
| Christopher D. Bojrab | 2004-2005 |
| Frederick P. Rauscher | 2005-2006 |
| David L. Wagner | 2006-2007 |
| Donald P. Hay | 2007-2008 |
| Kelda H. Walsh | 2008-2009 |
| Andrew L. Morrison | 2009-2010 |
| David R. Diaz | 2010-2011 |

Manufactured By:    RR Donnelley
                    Momence, IL  USA
                    December, 2010